The Investigator's Guide to
Clinical Research
Third Edition

Dr. David Ginsberg

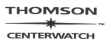
THOMSON

CENTERWATCH

THOMSON

CENTERWATCH™

The Investigator's Guide to Clinical Research – Third Edition
by Dr. David Ginsberg

Book Editor	**Publisher**	**Design**
Whitney Allen	Ken Getz	Paul Gualdoni

ISBN 1-930624-30-1

To my parents Anna and Samuel
without whose support I would not have gone into medicine,

To my wife Myrna
without whose support I would not have written this book,

And to our children Joshua, Alison, Jeffrey, Jonathan and Jenna,
without whose company I would not have enjoyed doing so nearly as much.

CONTENTS

Contents

Instructions for Obtaining Continuing Medical Education Credit

This book has been planned and produced in accordance with the Essentials and Standards of the Accreditation Council for Continuing Medical Education (ACCME).

With the purchase of the book, the owner is eligible to take an exam and receive four hours of Category 1 credit. The exam and instructions are available through the following web site:

www.centerwatch.com/bookstore/pubs_profs_invguide.html

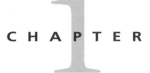

Should You Become a Clinical Investigator?

- Will You Enjoy It?
- Will it be Good for Your Patients?
- Are There Substantial Safety Risks for Patients?
- Will Participation in Clinical Research Inhibit the Growth of Your Practice?
- Will You Expose Your Practice to Legal Liabilities?

You are likely hearing more and more about clinical research. It seems as if every time you turn to a newspaper, radio or television, there is an advertisement for patients to enter a clinical trial. Each week, you probably are questioned by at least a few patients about the benefit of some experimental drug that they are sure will be the answer to their needs.

Americans are being inundated with information about promising new drugs. It is indeed an age in which we believe in the potential of modern medicine to resolve all our physical and emotional ills, if not immediately, then in the near future.

We are becoming used to hearing about experimental drugs and the protocols required for their development. Indeed, increasing numbers of our colleagues are conducting clinical trials. In 1990, there were only about 5,000 physicians and pharmacists who conducted a clinical trial of a new drug. This year, more like 50,000 medical professionals have assumed a role as principal investigator in an experimental drug trial. Clearly, the number of professionals participating in clinical trials is exploding, along with the number of patients in clinical trials and the overall number of trials.

Today, there are more drugs in the developmental pipeline than ever before and more individual trials are being conducted as part of the New Drug Application (NDA) than ever before. An average of about 80 trials are incorporated in the NDA annually, a number that increases each year. The sizes of studies are increasing, requiring many more patients than previously sought. Also, and perhaps most important, a new trend utilizes large, post-approval, surveillance protocols to expand knowledge of the product both for additional safety and marketing information.

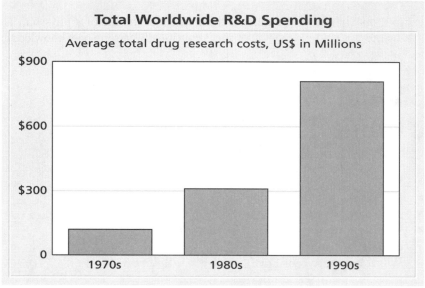

Source: Tufts University

The dramatic increases attest to the opportunities for the novice investigator to become involved in clinical research. However, it is also important to understand that today, many medical professionals as well as entrepreneurs with business backgrounds are exploring this opportunity. In fact, for a few years, many site management organizations (SMOs) were the darlings of the venture capitalists. Also, many practice management organizations, hospital chains and academic institutions are seeking portions of this lucrative pie. This phenomenon is not limited to the United States but is being explored in every corner of the globe. Even the Chinese government has enacted laws that make it difficult to market a new drug in that country without having some of the investigation work done by government-owned research centers.

Because of managed care and other significant changes in the medical environment, physicians today are faced with stagnating, or even decreasing, incomes. Frequently, they are losing some of their control over medical decisions because of oversight from managed care organizations and insurance companies. As a result, an increasing number of physicians are viewing clinical research as an opportunity that can provide both supplemental income and a new intellectual challenge.

Before diving into a detailed discussion about how to become a successful investigator, there are several critical questions you need to ask:

Will You Enjoy It?

One of the reasons that most people become physicians is that they love to learn. Probably one of the most exciting times in the life of a physician is during medical school when he or she is continually gaining new knowledge and being exposed to new technology. But even in medical school, when you devote 100% of your time to learning, it is impossible to keep up with the remarkable expansion in medical science. However, since few of us have the luxury of remaining a student our entire career, most of us become increasingly obsolete from the very day we leave our training programs. This is particularly true for physicians who are not associated with academic institutions and also for primary care physicians simply because of the overwhelming wealth of information. Many of us struggle futilely against this obsolescence by finding ways to work with students, interns and residents. Frequently though, the trainees become the teachers because they bring a wealth of new experiences and exposures to the table, while we in practice tend to rehash the same experiences over and over again.

Many of us read obsessively, listen to audio tapes in our cars, and attend conferences when we can afford it. Despite all our efforts, we feel increasingly distant from the cutting edge of medical science. Even though we become aware of new drugs and medical development, we are frequent-

 A Continuing Education

A few years ago, I conducted a number of studies involving a new class of antidepressants (serotonin antagonists). As part of the protocol, I was required to administer Hamilton Depression Scales to patients enrolling into the study. During the investigator meeting, I received fairly extensive training in this procedure. I was able to apply this diagnostic test to patients in the study, and also made it a regular part of my routine medical practice.

In summary, through these trials, I received early and extensive training in the use of a new class of drugs; I improved my normal practice procedures; and I impressed the heck out of my resident. Finally, because I enrolled a large number of patients in one of the trials, I was asked to participate in the writing of the clinical paper and later, I was recruited to speak to many local groups of family doctors about this study.

ly reluctant to utilize this knowledge. There is a great distance between understanding that a new product is out there and actually prescribing a product that might expose a patient to new, potential hazards. We might be more familiar with an older product that works, perhaps not as well as the new one is claimed to, but of which we are comfortably able to recognize and deal with any adverse responses.

If you want to remain close to medical science and to the development of new drugs and devices that correspond to the way you practice, then clinical research may be both emotionally and intellectually satisfying. At times, you can have the exciting experience of being involved in truly innovative products that are breakthroughs in treating specific diseases. When this happens, you feel that you have contributed to medicine and to the general welfare in a way that is difficult to replicate. But, value can even be derived from testing a "me too" product or a third or fourth medication in a class, a more probable scenario. It is likely, that if you become involved in a trial, you will be educated and ultimately become very much more effective in the treatment of that specific disease entity. By participating in a trial you will learn basic pathology and pharmacology as you explore the mechanism of action of that specific drug. Also, you will come into contact with experts in the field who will instruct you in their methodology in treatment, and you will probably utilize, as part of the study, the most modern and specific method of measurement to assess both efficacy and toxicity. All these things are applicable and will improve your current techniques in treating your other, non-study patients.

Another benefit to becoming involved in clinical research is becoming an author of the trial report. Frequently, investigators who have successfully enrolled a large number of qualified patients are asked to help write the trial results in a scholarly medical journal. This, of course, leads to many speaking opportunities, some of which are a natural result of the publication and others of which are because of promotion by the pharmaceutical company. Public speaking, by the way, can also result in some healthy stipends and a nice supplement to your income in and of itself. However, the chief joy comes from the fact that your colleagues perceive you to have some specific expertise. It is very gratifying to be able to introduce something in the way of new information to your comrades-in-arms.

Your accreditation board may accept publishing in journals and attending start-up or post-trial meetings as continuing medical education credits. The same is true of those lectures you deliver.

Will it be Good for Your Patients?

Over the last 20 years, there has been an increasing and accelerating acceptance of clinical trials by both the public and the medical community. Prior to this time, however, the general public viewed clinical research with a skeptical eye. Much of the skepticism was fueled by two well-publicized scandals. In the 1960s, in what came to be known as the Jewish Chronic Hospital Scandal, a physician conducted immune system research at a Brooklyn hospital, injecting live cancer cells into elderly persons without their consent. Most physicians responsible for the care of these patients were not consulted and knew nothing of this research. Then came the revelations of the Tuskegee study. The Tuskegee observational study began in the 1930s and continued for more than 40 years. During this period, more than 400 African-Americans were left to undergo the ravages of syphilis, despite the ready availability of antibiotic treatments. When the details of the experiment became public in the 1970s, some of the patients still had not been treated. Ultimately President Clinton apologized on behalf of the United States government to the victims of this study.

In 1975, along with 34 other countries, we in the United States signed the Helsinki Accords. The Accords include the World Medical Association Declaration of Helsinki and recommendations guiding the treatment of patients in biomedical research and have been updated several times. These recommendations include specific mandates involving consenting patients and the treatment and safety of patients, and generally outlines a moral approach to the conduct of clinical trials. It places the responsibility for the appropriate conduct of a trial and the satisfying of these principles squarely on the physician's shoulders. It is worth familiarizing yourself with this document, which is appended to this book and is also included in most clinical research protocols.

In the 1980s, public opinion concerning clinical trials began to shift. To a large extent, change was triggered by the AIDS community. AIDS patients actively sought to enroll in clinical trials in order to gain access to investigation therapies that offered them their only hope. As we have now seen, clinical trials did indeed provide many people infected with HIV early access to a new class of drugs – the protease inhibitors – that are effective in control

 The Patient is Always Right

Mrs. C enters a trial for her severe osteoarthritis of the hip and was randomized to receive a placebo treatment arm. During the course of the therapy, her arthritis improved but Mrs. C developed a rash that she insisted was a result of the placebo. The placebo was an inert substance, and, it seemed to me, highly unlikely to be responsible for her diffuse and itchy rash, but I could not come up with an alternative explanation. Mrs. C was certain about the etiology, however, and also insisted that the sponsoring company pay for her multiple visits to dermatologists as well as the therapies she was taking for a nonspecific allergic dermatitis. I referred her to the medical monitor at the company who denied her treatment stating categorically that this was not a result of the placebo drug. As a result of this incident, Mrs. C and her family left my practice.

ling the AIDS virus. In a very real sense, the opportunity to participate in these trials saved subjects' lives, and while this had occasionally happened in previous types of trials, the exposure here was enormous.

With their increasing visibility, clinical trials began to become less frightening. Since the 1980s, it has become very common for people, as they navigate through their daily routines, to encounter opportunities to participate. Trials are advertised on television, radio, billboards, newspapers and over the Internet. Clinical research has moved from the exotic to the commonplace.

A positive attitude toward clinical research is now becoming common among patient groups of all types. Many cancer patients regularly explore clinical research trials as part of their evaluation of treatment options. When Rhone Poulenc Rorer conducted trials of Rilutek for amyotrophic lateral sclerosis, so many patients clamored to get into the research trials that Rhone Poulenc had to hold a lottery to select those that would be enrolled. By the way, when this drug was approved in 1995, Rilutek became the first treatment available that effectively slowed the course of the disease.

 ## A Draw for Patients

A few years ago, when Imetrex was being tested for the treatment of migraines, I was fortunate to be chosen as an investigational site. There was great interest from patients suffering from this frequently disabling disorder. Within days of posting a notice of the study on my office bulletin board, I had a long list of potential subjects. Glaxo, the manufacturer of the drug, also released my name to the medical community as one of the investigators of this innovative drug. Consequently, my phone began ringing off the wall with requests from other physicians requesting that I include members of their families in the study. Eventually, I decided to take eight of the sixteen slots I had available and offer them to my colleagues. I distinctly remember one physician's wife driving from her home near Pittsburgh to my office near Philadelphia (across the entire state of Pennsylvania) twice a month.

The shift in public opinion has led groups lobbying for women, children and the elderly to push the Food and Drug Administration (FDA) and the National Institutes of Health (NIH) for greater access to clinical research. Both the FDA and NIH have now implemented guidelines designed to ensure that all people, including women, children, the elderly and minorities, have the opportunity to participate in clinical research. Recently, the FDA has been very concerned about the lack of drug testing in the pediatric population. It has begun to encourage pharmaceutical companies to test in this segment of the population by actually increasing the length of time by up to six months that a company has the exclusive rights to market a particular product. You may not think that this is a significant incentive, but if you consider that an innovative drug may bring in revenue of between one and five million dollars per day, you begin to see the magnitude of this change.

There is currently some speculation that the same incentive may be applied to testing drugs targeted to minorities as well.

It is clear that public interest in clinical research is increasing. This can be measured by the increase in activity seen on the Internet. For example, the CenterWatch Clinical Trials Listing Service is a web site where many pharmaceutical companies and contract research organizations (CROs) list trials for which they are currently recruiting. This site also serves the same function for the NIH. The number of visits to this site is increasing at a substantial rate, and currently there are more than 500,000 such visits each month. These visits are usually made by individuals seeking to find trials and physicians in their regions who are conducting the trials in which they are interested in participating. The use of the Internet, by the way, is creating some significant dilemmas for foreign regulatory bodies who have yet to deal with the unlimited and global access the Internet provides.

Clinical trials are also frequently mentioned in the press. Invariably, there are articles in the medical or science sections of the newspapers and frequent discussions on every talk show from "Good Morning America" to local public access channels.

As a physician who conducts clinical research, you will be providing your patients with additional treatment options. This can be vitally important for people with life-threatening or chronic diseases. It also can be of major importance to those individuals who simply have not found appropriate medical solutions to more mundane illnesses. For example, patients often cannot tolerate the current best therapy because of idiosyncratic reactions, side effects or allergies. The ability to offer all these individuals something new and potentially effective is a significant accomplishment. So, in a very real sense, a physician engaged in clinical research is providing his or her patient with the opportunity for improved medical care. Your patients will view you as a physician who is on the cutting edge of medicine.

There is another reason that becoming involved in clinical research can be good for your patients. Many people today have inadequate health insurance or none at all. For some people, the only way they can afford medical treatment for their chronic conditions and ailments is to enroll in clinical trials. Volunteers in clinical trials are not charged for either the medication or treatment, if it specifically involves the indications relevant to the trial. But it is also not unusual for patients' other illnesses or minor complaints to be treated at no charge if they are participating in a trial. In fact, it is a good business practice to reward those patients who participate in this manner because they are actually allowing you to make more in the way of income from their participation than you would normally earn from conventionally treating them.

Small stipends are frequently paid to patients who participate in clinical trials in the United States. In general, these are earmarked to reimburse patients for their time and travel. It is important that these stipends not be large enough to be considered coercive, and if they approach that level, your institutional review board (IRB) will disallow them. However, if the patient

New Drug Therapies (2001)

Disease	Drug Name	Date of Approval
rheumatoid arthritis	Remicade	January 2001
osteoarthritis	Supartz	January 2001
depression	Remeron SolTab	January 2001
breast cancer	Femara	January 2001
osteoarthritis	Supartz	January 2001
invasive aspergillosis	Cancidas	January 2001
hepatitis C	Peg-Intron	January 2001
depression	Prozac Weekly	February 2001
schizophrenia	Ziprasidone	February 2001
chronic periodontitis	Arestin	February 2001
periodontal disease	Periostat	February 2001
Alzheimer's	Reminyl	February 2001
migraine	Zomig-ZMT	February 2001
vaginal yeast infections	Monistat 3 Combination Pack	February 2001
asthma	Foradil	February 2001
glaucoma	Lumigan	March 2001
glaucoma	Travatan	March 2001
cytomegalovirus (CMV) retinitis	Valcyte	March 2001
tinea	Lamisil Solution	March 2001
gastroesophageal reflux disease	Protonix	March 2001
bronchospasm associated with COPD	DuoNeb Inhalation Solution	March 2001
cold and allergy	Tavist Allergy/Sinus/ Headache	March 2001
hyperphosphetemia	PhosLo	April 2001
attention deficit/ hyperactivity disorder	Metadate CD	April 2001
migraine	Axert	May 2001
acne	Finvein	May 2001
thyroid replacement therapy	Levoxyl	May 2001
hepatitis	Twinrix	May 2001
contraception	Yasmin	May 2001
leukemia	Campath	May 2001
chronic myeloid leukemia	Gleevec	May 2001
colorectal cancer	Xeloda	May 2001
acne vulgaris	Estrostep	July 2001
hepatitis C	Rebetol	July 2001
growth failure	Genotropin	July 2001

* Patients in clinical trials were able to gain access to these promising therapies years before they were approved by the FDA.

is devoting a large amount of time to his or her participation in the trial and also undergoing time-consuming and uncomfortable procedures, these stipends can add up to a significant amount. For example, it is usually considered appropriate to reimburse a patient $150 or $200 for undergoing a gastroscopic examination as part of a trial, and there might be multiple procedures in any given trial. In other countries there is great variation in the ability of investigators to compensate patients. In some places (i.e., Spain or Belgium), it is forbidden.

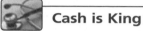 ## Cash is King

Jenna was 10 years old and had agreed to participate in a trial for a new spray analgesic to palliate her sore throat. She performed her tasks well but during the hour she had to remain in the office, she asked several times about the $25 stipend, which was promised at the end of the trial. It was our policy, whenever possible, to reward those patients who participated in clinical trials immediately on completion. Jenna was presented with her check at the termination of the trial but refused to accept it and insisted that I be called into the examination room along with her mother, who was in the waiting room. Jenna then confronted me with her demand that she be paid in cash. This crisis was resolved by a swift raid on the petty cash drawer and thus terminated to everyone's satisfaction.

These stipends, along with free medical care, can provide significant benefit to patients living on marginal incomes and frequently allow for these people to receive comprehensive medical care in addition to access to some very promising therapies.

It is important that you, as an individual who is considering involvement with clinical trials, understand both the positive and negative ramifications of your involvement. In a study done for the NIH in 1997, R. Mechanic dubbed a potential negative issue as "the zone of uncertainty." In the way of background, patients participating in clinical research are guaranteed treatment of any side effects or complications that occur as a result of their direct participation in that trial. This is a necessary element of the consent form. "The zone of uncertainty" occasionally occurs when there is an attempt to determine whether a particular complication is a result of the trial or a natural course of that patient's pathologic process. For example, if a patient is entered into an angina trial and suffers an exacerbation that requires his or her hospitalization (while beginning to be treated with an experimental drug as opposed to standard therapy), then who is responsible for the cost of that hospitalization: the pharmaceutical company or the patient's insurance company? It is possible for the patient to be caught in the middle here, and he or she might have to involve an attorney to rectify this situation. Again this is a rare occurrence.

"The zone of uncertainty" issue evolved as a result of managed care. Prior to the current age, insurance companies seldom knew if their patients were involved in clinical trials. Today it is likely a patient being treated outside of the normal paradigm and referral patterns sanctioned by the HMO will be quickly discovered.

Clinical trials can be good for your patients, if you bear in mind some important axioms. The first axiom for all clinical investigators must be to do no harm. It is most important that, in your medical opinion, there are no significant dangers to which you would expose your patients unnecessarily. And this, of course, includes any risk involved in stopping that patient's current therapy. Clearly, though, everything is relative. In a life-threatening illness, more risk might still be well within the realm of acceptability.

A second axiom is that a patient should never in any way be coerced into a clinical trial. A clinical trial must be presented in a fair and balanced way and the decision to enter must be left to the patient, who needs to be free from both overt and covert influences. As that patient's physician, you must refrain from allowing your own desires to inadvertently influence the patient. Remember that you are an authority figure, and that frequently, patients will act out of a desire to please you rather than in a way that they perceive as in their own best interests.

A third important axiom is that the patient must have a complete understanding of the risks, benefits and requirements of a clinical trial. It is important that the consent form (which delineates safety, visit requirements, etc.) be reviewed in detail by the investigator at a level that is compatible with that patient's language skills and intellect. It is also worth presenting this information to other members of the patient's family, so that everyone has a clear understanding of the situation. In fact, it has always been my practice to have a patient's family member witness his or her signature on the consent form.

Are There Substantial Safety Risks for Patients?

You and your patients may be concerned about patient safety issues. What are the risks associated with volunteering for a clinical study? There can be risks, but the research process is designed to minimize them.

Most investigators become involved in conducting phase II through phase IV trials and rarely do phase I. There will be further discussion about all the trial phases in chapter one. However, prior to phase I where a drug is tested for the first time in healthy humans, all products undergo extensive animal testing. So, by the time a drug reaches phase II tests, much has been learned about the drug's toxicity, half-life and potential side effects.

The general intention of phase II trials is to further expand safety and dosing knowledge. Therefore, an investigator involving himself or herself in phase III trials can be assured of much more information regarding these parameters. And, phase III trials are the earliest phase of trials in which practically all clinical investigators will become involved. It is extremely rare for any novice or inexperienced investigator to be considered for any early or phase II work.

As an investigator, you will receive a protocol and a drug manual. The drug manual delineates all the relevant knowledge that has been accumulated about the drug being tested. It includes animal data as well as information on phase I testing and any previous phase II and phase III trials done anywhere in the world. A copy of this manual, along with the protocol, must be forwarded to your IRB prior to approval of the trial. It is vital that you, as an investigator, read this manual carefully so you can become familiar with any potential problems or side effects discovered earlier in the drug development process. Not only does this information impinge upon your decision to take the trial, but it makes you aware of what problems to look for as the trial progresses. Please remember that you must be comfortable with the risks and benefits to your patients in the trial. If you are worried about undue hazards or side effects that seem too severe to justify, then you should not take this trial. It is impossible for an investigator to function effectively under these types of circumstances. So, always remember that you are the final judge of what is appropriate and what is not.

 ## Adverse Events

I agreed to become an investigator for a trial treating patients suffering from nosocomial pneumonia with an antibiotic that was marketed in an oral form but now was being tested in an intravenous form for serious and life-threatening illnesses. I was very comfortable doing this, because I previously participated in the phase II and phase III testing of the oral preparation and had no problems. Also, the medication had been on the market for two years and hundreds of thousands of doses had been consumed. Unfortunately, the first two patients that I treated suffered hepatic and renal failure within five days of entering into the study. The study was stopped, and after an FDA and sponsor investigation, it was determined that the test drug was the cause. Retrospective analysis of the marketed oral preparation was done, and it was determined that there were multiple incidents of liver and renal failure in the general public who had been exposed to the oral preparation. The drug was withdrawn from the marketplace and many lives were saved.

Most clinical trials you become involved with will not be on "first in the class" products, but on "me too" drugs. While this creates less interest for the investigator, it adds a great margin of comfort because a similar product has already been marketed, and the side effect and safety profile will probably be rather similar.

It can be argued that patients in clinical trials are actually safer than patients not in clinical trials who are taking the same or similar products. This is because patients in clinical trials are much better monitored than those who are not. Trials require many more visits to the physician than what is typical in routine practice and also, in general, much more frequent testing than would normally be done. Also, the clinical tests and parameters utilized are frequently at the highest level of technology available. For example, how many of your hypertensive patients have three 24-hour blood pressure monitors applied in a six-month period?

Frequently, because of the thoroughness of the examinations required by clinical trials, serious and silent coexisting disorders are uncovered. During my experience conducting clinical trials, I have uncovered three malignancies only because of the extensive testing required by the protocol. In two of the cases, the patient's life was saved.

When considering involvement in clinical trials, it is important to step back for a moment and to consider participation from a different perspective. It has been stated that the administration of one million doses of a medication is required before an adequate side effect profile is developed. In most instances, a medication is released on the market after administration of several thousand doses or less. It is clear from the frequent withdrawal of marketed medications that many people are in danger of suffering untoward and potentially serious side effects from many medications that are assumed to be safe because they have received FDA approval. It is important to remember that every time someone takes a medication, whether it be approved, over the counter, herbal or as part of an experimental protocol, there are potential dangers.

This isn't to minimize concerns about patients in clinical trials experiencing adverse events. Research trials are designed to produce a profile of the drug's side effects as well as the drug's efficacy. The close monitoring of patients in clinical trials, however, ensures that physician, patient and coordinator will pay close attention to any adverse effects. This is a crucial safety factor.

In addition to concerns about the possible side effects of the study drug, an investigator also needs to consider the risk posed by the use of either a placebo or another active substance used as a standard or comparative agent. A patient who receives a placebo (inactive substance) must not be placed in a compromised position as a result of not receiving treatment. Also, a comparative agent must be one that meets current standards of care, and this should be in keeping with the standard that is acceptable in the region where you practice. Frequently, acceptable standards of care vary between the United States and Europe. If your protocol was designed by a European company, their assumptions of what medication is appropriate might be quite correct in Europe but not the standard of care here. Legally and ethically, you are judged by local standards.

All studies must be approved by an IRB that looks closely at the appropriateness of using a placebo and also at the choice of comparative agents. An IRB will not allow a trial to be placebo-controlled if this creates significant risk to the subjects in that trial. IRBs function as "watchdogs" and sit in judgment of the morality and risk to patients. They are structured to contain sufficient scientific and medical expertise to protect those who enter as subjects in clinical research and who do not have sufficient knowledge to protect themselves.

You also will find that a placebo can be a wonderful "drug" for your patients as it frequently is highly effective and has minimal side effects. It is interesting to note that a placebo is an effective therapy in almost 30% of all hypertensive patients entering a clinical trial. It is also effective in many other conditions including anxiety, tension headaches, muscular spasms, etc. In clinical trials, patients frequently do well because of the tender loving care they receive as participants. A strong supportive relationship frequently develops between the office staff and trial participants. Often the study coordinator assumes a role somewhere between best friend and therapist, and this relationship translates into overall improvement in the patient's health.

Another potential benefit to the patient is the withdrawal of a patient from his or her current therapeutic regime. There are potential advantages in giving some patients drug holidays. It became apparent to me, while participating in hypertension trials, that many patients, when removed from their drugs, remained normotensive. In my experience, this occurred in up to 20 percent of those who withdrew from ongoing therapy. Many of these patients have been treated for years, and I had considered them stable because of their medications. Actually they had, for some reason, returned to normotensive status. This impressed me so much that I instituted a policy to slowly and carefully withdrawal all hypertensive medications, from mild to moderately hypertensive patients, once a year.

It is your decision regarding the appropriateness of any protocol, including the decision about the comparative agent or placebo. Yours is the final say as to whether you are comfortable and whether your patients will participate. It is all right to say no, and most individuals on the sponsor's side will respect your integrity. After all, you are placing these issues before a lucrative contract. In fact, sometimes saying no is a very effective strategy because the sponsor will frequently return to you when they discover that your logic and reasoning is valid

No pharmaceutical company will penalize an investigator for deciding not to participate in a protocol as long as the investigator decides when initially presented with the protocol, not after signing a contract. It is a mistake not to explore up front any concerns you may have about a trial. If you are worried about safety issues, it is unlikely that you will pursue enrollment in the trial the way it needs to be done to have a successful outcome. Consequently, you will fail and not meet your commitment to the sponsor – an outcome that is much worse than if you had never taken the trial at all.

Will Participation in Clinical Research Inhibit the Growth of Your Practice?

Most of us have worked very hard to build and grow a practice, so concern about the effect that clinical research might have on an ongoing practice is appropriate. No one should do anything to jeopardize something of such great value without prolonged and careful consideration.

When considering venturing into the clinical research world, your patients' perceptions are an important issue but your associates', partners' and staff's receptivity are also important. It is clear that when you introduce an endeavor with such enormous potential into a stable organization, there is a strong possibility of disrupting functions. You must explore all potential changes in advance. These include changes in work scheduling, coverage, measurements of productivity and income.

If you don't plan out an appropriate structure up front, then it is likely that this pursuit will end in disaster. Many practices have been torn apart when one partner becomes increasingly involved in research to the detriment of his or her regular and customary duties. Also, when these activities result in additional cash, there are frequently problems because little thought was given, up front, to alignment of rewards and labor. New relationships, mechanisms and paradigms must be worked out between the partners in a practice. Extra cash is always helpful to a medical practice, but dividing the money is frequently contentious, particularly when one party feels that he or she has been predominately responsible for the windfall.

In the past, those physicians who chose to indulge in the pursuit of clinical research frequently found that their colleagues did not understand what they were doing. The other physicians in the area assumed that this was a scheme to move their patients to the researcher's own practice, and the fact that the subjects were not charged heightened their suspicions. The further removed a physician was from academic centers, the more of a factor this was. Today this response seems less likely as more of the medical community is aware of clinical trials but still, you must be prepared for a negative reaction particularly if you are the first in the region to get your feet wet.

Interestingly enough, most physicians who have gotten involved in clinical research will attest to the fact that clinical research has actually helped to build their practice. Physicians in clinical research often find that their reputations are enhanced in their local communities. They are perceived as being on the "cutting edge" of medical knowledge and as having access to the most innovative and modern therapies. Frequently, practice doctors who do research find that they achieve a high profile through positive stories in the press and through recruitment efforts either sponsored by the physician or by the sponsoring company. For example, one recruitment strategy for an influenza vaccine trial might be to give lectures at senior citizen activity centers. Clearly, you would gain a reputation as an expert on this disease in your community and probably, as a result of your education in conjunction with the trial, this perception would be correct.

As a principal investigator, some time and travel will be required. First, you must educate yourself about the process and the responsibilities of doing trials. You must understand and supervise each trial, interact with the IRB, develop budgets, deal with audits and inspections, and perform other duties. If structured appropriately, this should not be an overwhelming amount of your time but it does require attention. Doing clinical trials is not a hands-off activity. Of course, the income produced from these activities will far exceed what you can do through routine practice. However, as a group, your practice must deal with fair divisions of money and labor. The principal investigator will need to be covered when he or she attends start-up meetings, resulting in an increased workload for the others. Your partners will need to be compensated for their extra work.

You will change all the dynamics and interpersonal relationships in your office when you introduce specific personnel such as study coordinators. The current staff might perceive these changes as increasing their workloads without increasing their compensation. For example, your receptionist might consider that his or her new requirement to get a separate appointment book for each study coordinator and the need to schedule monitoring visits from the company are simply extra burdens. On the other hand, if this additional work is accompanied by additional perks or the opportunity to earn additional income, he or she might be the coordinators' best advocate.

Your nursing staff might perceive your coordinator as a new elitist addition to the office and their status might be threatened by the introduction of a better-trained and paid individual. They may find themselves relegated to a lower rung in the new hierarchy. However, this can be mitigated if the coordinator has an appropriate attitude and also, perhaps, lends a hand to the office staff during peak times.

Specific ways to deal with these issues will be discussed in later chapters.

Any physician considering becoming involved in clinical research needs to weigh all the pros and cons. Clinical research can clearly help a physician rediscover the intellectual joys of medicine. You will feel the rewards of becoming part of a community of researchers. You will, on occasion, have the opportunity to contribute to the advancement of medical therapeutics. There are also definite financial advantages because clinical research has the potential to develop revenues that are hard to duplicate through any other medical endeavor. However, on the down side, your rewards will be directly proportional to the degree to which you involve yourself. This is not to say that research needs to ultimately occupy a major slice of your time. On the contrary, you can be quite successful by allocating 15% or 20% of your time to it. But, at the front end, if you do not understand the regulatory, scientific and fiscal components, you will do it poorly and also not achieve your best financial success.

It is important that you understand that this activity is a business enterprise and the more you utilize good business practices, the more likely your business will flourish. It will require appropriate structuring, attention and fiscal support. This is not a passive activity, and you must be prepared to devote some of your time and energy to learning about all aspects of this business and the proper way to conduct trials. Also, you need to adequately capitalize it. This activity, in general, does not require a great deal of money, but one of the major errors people make is the undercapitalization of this enterprise. You need to think about all these issues before deciding if clinical research is truly the right path for you. I think involvement in clinical research is well worth it but you must make your own decision.

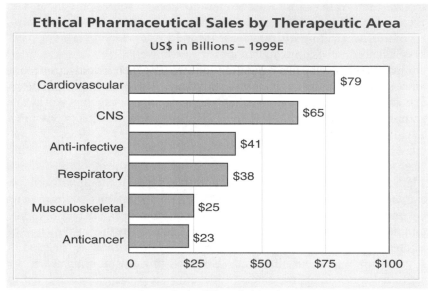

Ethical Pharmaceutical Sales by Therapeutic Area
US$ in Billions – 1999E

Therapeutic Area	US$ in Billions
Cardiovascular	$79
CNS	$65
Anti-infective	$41
Respiratory	$38
Musculoskeletal	$25
Anticancer	$23

Source: Dorland Biomedical Database

Will You Expose Your Practice to Legal Liabilities?

A commonly asked question is whether clinical research will increase your malpractice exposure or increase malpractice insurance premiums. To my knowledge, this is not the case, but it would be wise for all those considering involvement to contact their insurance carrier. It is, in fact, my impression that involvement in clinical research decreases exposure, but this is dependent upon the investigator being diligent in adherence to the protocol. If you stray from the sanctioned pathway, you might find yourself on your own. For example, if you ignore inclusion and exclusion criteria or admit a subject who clearly is a protocol violation and that subject has a mishap because of this, you might very well find yourself out on a limb.

Whenever a patient enters a clinical trial, he or she must sign the consent form. As long as consent is obtained properly and the form is designed to meet good clinical practice (GCP) standards, it provides a good deal of legal protection to both the researcher and the pharmaceutical company. The patient, through his or her signature, understands the potential risks, and therefore, assumes a measure of responsibility.

A pharmaceutical sponsor will normally indemnify the investigator against lawsuits. Again, this indemnification is contingent upon the investigator following GCP practices and the protocol. If, for some reason, indemnification is not included in the initial contract, it normally will be supplied upon request. I think that it is important to be indemnified but I have some questions about the ultimate value because if push came to shove, an investigator might have to sue a pharmaceutical company to enforce it. To place this discussion in context, I believe that sponsoring companies will, in general, fight to the death to protect their investigators. If a pharmaceutical company ever developed a reputation for throwing their investigators to the wolves, that company might as well shut down. The most important determinate of success in today's marketplace is the pipeline of new products a company develops. Without ongoing positive relationships with investigators, these drugs could not be developed.

Another point is that plaintiffs in a lawsuit, although they will sue everyone involved, are generally after those with the deepest pockets. This clearly is the sponsoring company.

To my knowledge, it is extremely rare for any clinical investigator to be sued. In my experience and after questioning many active investigators, I was unable to uncover one case. Again, this is not to say that it hasn't happened or can't happen, but it would be a rare event.

A different issue, but one that needs to be discussed, is fraud. On a rare occasion, and primarily for financial reasons, an investigator or someone employed by an investigator acts in bad faith and makes up data or even entire patients. This, of course, can result not only in financial ramifications but also in criminal charges. Those who do it and are caught wind up on the FDA's blacklist and are restricted from future participation in clinical trials. This type of behavior always amazes me because clinical research is so lucrative when done in the right way.

 ## Safer Way to Practice

When I began doing clinical research I called my malpractice carrier to ask about any increased risk. It took several days for them to get back to me but when they did, the gentleman on the phone told me that their preference was that I do only clinical research and stop practicing medicine outside of that context.

Recently, there has been some news about insider trading by clinical investigators. A few physicians have actually suffered criminal and civil penalties because of stock purchases they, their friends and relatives have made. An investigator is always required to sign confidentiality agreements, so when someone does this sort of thing, he or she is flying strictly on his or her own. An investigator is entitled to act only on information that is in the public domain. If you hear something about the new product on which you are working on the radio or while listening to the Financial Network, you are entitled to purchase or sell stock based on that information. You, however, are not entitled to act on information that accrues to you as a result of your work that is supposed to be conducted in a confidential manner.

The Clinical Development Process

- The Pipeline of New Drug Therapies
- Drug Development Growth Areas
- The Drug Discover Process
- The Clinical Trials Phases

I
n medical school, little attention is given to the drug development process. Drug development is covered, if at all, in a superficial manner. Consequently most of us go on to practice with only minimal understanding of the process. Drug development is, for most physicians, the same as a computer. We all generally know how to use it. The rest is a deep and murky mystery.

If you choose to pursue clinical trials, it is important that you gain a better understanding of the process. This will allow you to clearly see why some issues are of greater importance than others to the sponsors and the contract research organizations (CROs). It will help you appreciate exactly what is expected from a site.

The Pipeline of New Drug Therapies

In 1995, pharmaceutical and biotechnology companies had an estimated 5,800 compounds in development. By 1998, that number was closer to 11,000.

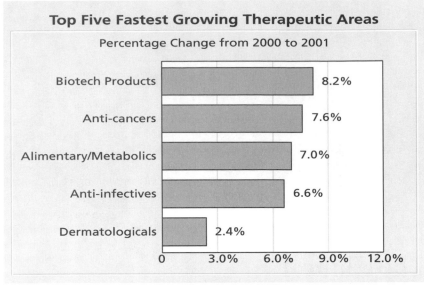

Top Five Fastest Growing Therapeutic Areas

Percentage Change from 2000 to 2001

- Biotech Products — 8.2%
- Anti-cancers — 7.6%
- Alimentary/Metabolics — 7.0%
- Anti-infectives — 6.6%
- Dermatologicals — 2.4%

(0   3.0%   6.0%   9.0%   12.0%)

Source: Pharmaprojects, 2001

However, between 1995 and 1997, the FDA approved only 123 drugs, an average of 70 new drug approvals per year. It is clear that the process of bringing a drug to market is risky, and there are many more failures than successes.

It typically takes a pharmaceutical company 10 years from the time a drug is first tested in humans to the time the FDA approves it. It is an incredibly expensive process, costing a company up to an estimated half a billion dollars.

The consequences of this huge cost and the long development time means that sponsoring companies must quickly recoup enormous amounts of money. Generally a company will have only seven years of exclusive rights to its developed product after it reaches the market. After drugs lose their patent protection, generic equivalents of the more common drugs can significantly erode market share.

A somewhat similar circumstance exists in "first of a class" products. The first of a new class of compounds always has a running start on the competition. The best of all worlds, of course, is to be the first of a new class and to have no competition at all. However, the usual scenario is a year or two at the most of this blissful existence. Every day, a drug having exclusivity in the marketplace can account for between one and five million dollars in sales.

The fiscal squeeze – growing research and development costs and increased competition for market share – has led pharmaceutical companies to aggressively strive to find ways to accelerate the clinical development process. Time is more important than cost, but cost counts, too.

These factors actually led to the development of the CROs. Because of the variable nature of the research pipeline, sponsoring companies can consistently save a lot of personnel costs by not staffing except for periods of

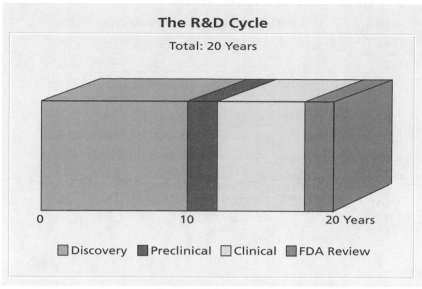

The R&D Cycle

Total: 20 Years

0   10   20 Years

☐ Discovery ■ Preclinical ☐ Clinical ■ FDA Review

Source: FDA, Tufts Center

peak need. Most companies staff to 75% of research needs or less. The remainder of the job is contracted out. CROs fit this need. Ideally, CROs would also be able to do the development job more quickly and more cleanly because it is the only thing they do. This has not proved to be the case. CROs seem to be just as cumbersome as the pharmaceutical companies for whom they work. However, a CenterWatch survey revealed that sponsoring companies hired CROs for 61% of their clinical development projects.

Drug Development Growth Areas

For an investigator, it is advantageous to know what drugs are in the development process and where they are in that process. This enables an investigator to be proactive in pursuit of trials in which he or she might be interested in participating. One way to do this is to subscribe to some of the industry publications that track this development process.

Several excellent sources include the Pink Sheet, CenterWatch monthly and weekly newsletters, R&D Directions magazine and Scrip Reports. The contact information for these publications can be found in the Industry Resources section of the appendix.

Drug research and development is constantly changing. Some therapeutic areas seem to come into favor as others go out. It is difficult to predict what tomorrow's hot areas will be, but today the areas in which the greatest amount of research is occurring include oncology, central nervous system and cardiovascular. Together, these account for about 35% of all trials.

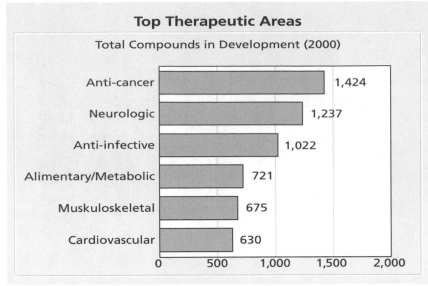

Source: Pharmaprojects, 2001

There also seems to have been a trend away from the common, mundane disorders to more "niche" diseases. Perhaps much of the low-hanging fruit has already been picked by the sponsoring companies. Despite this, there are still more than sufficient new products for application to the more common ills faced by mankind. In fact, the huge blockbuster drugs are those that address these common and mundane problems that so many of us just live with on a day-to-day basis. What this all means is that if your specialty training is in a current hot area, then you are in luck, and there will probably be a ton of work for you. In addition, if your specialty is primary care or a general medical field, there will always be plenty to keep you busy.

The Drug Discovery Process

Drug development is divided into phases I through IV. Frequently, there is no clear separation between the phases, but they should still be considered as general guidelines. In addition, some trials are classified as IIIB. This is a phase of development that occurs after the new drug application (NDA) is submitted but before approval has been issued by the FDA. With rare exceptions, a novice investigator should look to involve himself or herself in late phase clinical trials. The best opportunities are in phase III and phase IIIB trials. Phase IV, or post-approval, trials are increasingly frequent because the FDA more often requests post-approval, long-term surveillance trials. However, there is generally a huge difference between the complexity of a phase III and a phase IV trial. A phase III trial might have a case report form of 12 to 15 pages per visit with eight to 10 visits. The entire case report form for a phase IV trial might be two to five pages.

Also, in most pharmaceutical companies, phase I through phase III trials are run by the research division, and phase IV trials are run by the marketing division. An investigator's work with the marketing division frequently does not translate into credibility as a researcher.

Before a pharmaceutical company can begin testing a drug in humans, extensive laboratory and animal testing must be done. The pre-clinical testing provides the company's scientists with an understanding of the drug's biological activity, toxicity, half-life and some indication of potential side effects. By some estimates, fewer than 1% of drugs that enter pre-clinical testing are ever tested in humans.

To begin human testing, the pharmaceutical company must present this pre-clinical data to the FDA and detail its plans for clinical trials of the drug. This is called an "Investigational New Drug" application, and a lack of FDA response allows the process to go forward.

All trials are conducted with the tacit approval of the FDA and the active approval of an IRB. As previously mentioned in chapter one, the IRB is the moral and ethical watchdog of the clinical trial process. No trial can be conducted in the United States without the supervision of an IRB. We will discuss IRBs more in chapter nine under regulatory issues.

The Clinical Trial Phases

Clinical trials are divided into four phases with subdivisions of phase II and phase III into A and B, designating early and late phase trials. Each phase involves a progressively larger population of subjects.

Phase I trials are primarily concerned with assessing drug safety. Usually, these trials are done on small numbers of healthy young volunteers (24 to 100), who are paid for their participation. A typical trial would require that 24 subjects be admitted to a dedicated phase I unit for 24 hours. During that period, serum drug levels and chemical profiles would be drawn on an hourly basis. The phase I subject would be confined to the phase I unit for this period and would receive approximately $150 to $200 for his or her participation. Frequently, the study requires an additional 24-hour period two weeks from the first testing period. An exception to this rule of isolation is the many types of phase I vaccine studies that can readily be accomplished in an outpatient facility.

There are some individuals who make a career out of participating in phase I trials, despite the fact that regulations prohibit subjects from participating in two clinical trials within a 30-day period. However, in an area like Philadelphia, where there are multiple phase I units, if a subject was less than honest, he or she could be involved in a clinical trial every couple of days. A subject participating in multiple trials in a short period of time can create problems for data interpretation because some blood chemistry changes might be the residual effect of a previous trial but would be attributed to the current trial.

The Clinical Development Cycle

	Number of patients and type	Typical length	Percent of drugs successfully completing*
Phase I	20–100 healthy, normal patients	up to one year	70%
Phase II	Up to several hundred patients	1–2 years	50%
Phase III	Several hundred to several thousand patients	2–4 years	80%

Source: FDA, 2000

* These percentages depict the frequency with which investigational drugs pass through particular stages of testing. Thus of 100 investigational drugs that enter phase I testing, 70 will successfully go on to phase II. Of the 70 that enter phase II, 35 will successfully go on to phase III. Of the 35 that enter phase III, about 25 to 30 will successfully complete this stage of testing.

Phase I units are interesting places. Today, there are many commercial, free-standing phase I units. Some have even been set up in strip malls. Generally, though, the units include some recreational facilities for the subjects, a kitchen, barracks-like living facilities and tight security. It is worth visiting one if you can identify a unit in your region.

At the end of phase I trials, the pharmaceutical company should have a fairly clear understanding of a drug's absorption, metabolism and excretion. Any obvious problems with the drug should be revealed as well. About 70% of those drugs introduced into humans successfully complete phase I testing.

Phase II is usually the first time a drug is used in a population for which the treatment is intended. The entire population of patients tested in phase II is usually less than 1,000 patients. Phase II trials are primarily focused on safety, and efficacy is a secondary issue. Starting with phase II trials, the "gold standard" of clinical trials begins to appear. This is the double-blind, placebo-controlled trial. Double-blind means that neither the patient nor the physician knows whether the patient is receiving active medication. Placebo-controlled trials are most acceptable to the FDA for proof of effectiveness and safety of a drug, but placebo-control would never be expected when there were potential seriously detrimental effects to the patient. When a placebo is used, the investigator is always given access to a randomization code that, in case of emergency, could be broken to determine whether the patient was on the active drug. This code is either in the form of sealed envelopes or, today, in the form of a voice-activated telephone system that responds to the proper codes. As an investigator, it is very important that you not break this code unless absolutely necessary. During my involvement in several hundred trials, I only had to break the randomization code on three occasions.

Phase II trials are seldom awarded to new investigators, but as you develop experience in the field, there will be opportunities to participate at this level. Only about one-third of investigational drugs successfully complete phase I and phase II testing.

After a successful phase II trial, the pharmaceutical company has good evidence of drug safety and some preliminary evidence of efficacy. The sponsor should already have an understanding of the drug's side effect profile. Phase III trials build further upon this knowledge, with the emphasis shifting from safety to efficacy. Phase III studies involve several hundred to several thousand patients and usually have several separate phase III trials running concomitantly. Each phase III trial may involve 30 to 100 centers across the United States. Frequently, some of these trials may be placed in other countries if patients are more readily available in a different region of the world, or if pre-clinical trials aid in the approval process in a place where the company intends to market the drug.

Those phase III trials that are going to be used to support the NDA are critical to the submission process and are referred to as "pivotal" trials. Some phase III trials are part of the original plan, and others are developed to respond to questions that arise out of phase II trials. Another reason to do phase III trials is when an already approved product is seeking a new indication or new dosage form. Actually, this is a terrific type of scenario for a new investigator to become involved in, because he or she would be dealing with a product that has been on the market and probably has already been administered to hundreds of thousands of patients. This is a sure prescription for increasing your comfort level when beginning to navigate clinical research.

For pharmaceutical companies, the biggest hurdle to completing phase III trials is enrolling sufficient numbers of patients. Sponsors regularly identify poor patient enrollment as the number one reason that phase III trials are delayed or even fail. Over half the clinical trials started need to extend enrollment timelines and over one-third of the sites recruited fail to meet their targets. This is an increasingly critical issue because phase III trials are becoming larger and larger requiring more patients in each trial. Not only that, there are more and more phase III trials in each NDA. Interestingly, much of this need for more trials is in response to the sponsoring companies' attempt to answer questions that might be posed by regulatory bodies anywhere in the world. Also, in this highly competitive market, every advantage is sought for each new drug in order to promote it. This means that trials are being designed to try to explore any potential difference that might make this product stand out in its class.

It stands to reason that if one-third of the recruited sites fail to meet their enrollment goals, then there is a need for highly productive sites to over-enroll patients. This is potentially a great financial benefit for a good site. It is possible for a good site to count on doubling or even tripling its enroll-ment in the vast majority of studies. These additional patients prove to be the most lucrative because the system is already in place: the staff expends less time per patient because they know what they are doing, there are min-imal additional regulatory costs and hurdles, and the site doesn't have to go to the trouble of recruiting an additional trial.

Since 1985, the average number of patients per NDA has increased from 3,200 to more than 4,000. As I discussed in chapter one, the FDA is also urg-ing sponsors to test their investigational drugs on the full spectrum of prospective patients: men, women, children, the elderly and diverse ethnic groups. In fact, there has been recent legislation approved that extends patent protection by six months, if sponsoring companies agree to conduct pediatric trials of their new product.

The increasing patient requirement creates a wonderful opportunity for the novice investigator to secure a phase III grant. If you have the patients in large numbers, you have a resource that is clearly needed by sponsors. Also, if you have the type of relationship with your patients where they want to work with you, then you are an element in the drug approval process that is rare and valuable.

Sponsors and CROs also view phase III trials as much less scientifically demanding than phase II research. There are many more investigators in a phase III trial than in a phase II trial, so a poorly enrolling site does not have the same impact. Consequently, companies are much more willing to trust a novice investigator in phase III trials.

Once phase III testing is complete, the pharmaceutical company submits the NDA to the FDA and awaits approval. Because of new regulations that allow the sponsoring company to subsidize the approval process, this takes much less time than it used to. However, during this delay, the company con-tinues to explore research that will widen the scope of its product, increas-ingly demonstrate efficacy, and accomplish other goals. These trials are clas-sified as phase IIIB. This is another excellent place for the novice investiga-tor to become involved since the outcome of these trials does not affect the submission. So while these trials are still under the direction of the research division of the company, there is less pressure to use known investigators.

After approval comes phase IV. These studies bridge the gap between research and marketing. Today, they are more commonly requested by the FDA because it is clear it takes large numbers of doses to understand all the potential side effects of a drug. In fact, all major litigation involving phar-maceutical products has occurred in marketed drugs. Examples are the Redux phenomenon and the silicon breast implant. Today, there is a clear need for quality of life trials as well as comparisons to cost of treatment. These kinds of trials are mandated in Europe. Here in the United States, however, decided economic advantages must be demonstrated in order to capture a share of the market. Large-scale phase IV trials are an excellent way to introduce physicians to the use of a new product. Consequently, sponsors sometimes use the volume of prescriptions written to determine where and with whom they want to place these trials.

The rapid increase in the number of investigators competing for grants may seem daunting to the novice investigator. But this is an industry enjoying explosive growth. Also, few investigators do it really well. Most sites do not present the industry with the required outcome: adequate numbers of patients and clean data. Most sites do not facilitate the research process. This means most investigators do not make their site "user-friendly."

For any service business to succeed, both the process and the outcome must be good. Pharmaceutical employees and CRO employees must be accommodated in a manner that makes it easy for them to work with the site. They must not be subjected to procedural paradigms that annoy them or complicate their jobs. Little things like having a private phone line just for the use of the pharmaceutical company representative, accommodating appointments, and giving these folks a comfortable place to work ensures that the process at a site accommodates research. Fortunately for the novice investigator, very few sites or institutions have gone the distance to make sure both process and outcome are right. There is an incredible amount of room for an effective, consistent site that has good, accommodating processes in place. These issues will be expanded upon in future chapters.

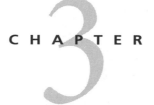

CHAPTER

The Grants Market

- Who Gets the Grants?
- Site Management Organizations (SMOs)
- Research Networks

There are several different ways that you can become involved in clinical research, and the financial opportunities will vary greatly depending on which route you take. You can choose involvement through site management organizations (SMOs), coordinator organizations, your academic affiliations or your practice management company. Or, you can move forward and develop your own research center, either in conjunction with your practice or as an independent free-standing site. As you would expect, the greater your commitment and involvement, the greater the financial rewards. This is also true of the risk. The more risk you assume, the greater the potential benefit. If you decide to plunge in completely and finance and develop your own site, the potential is enormous. This chapter will discuss what money is available to you through the grants market.

The amount spent by pharmaceutical and biotech companies on clinical trials is directly linked to their overall research and development expenditures. In fact, clinical trials are the single largest line item component of the budget, accounting for as much as half of all expenditures. During the past 15 years, industry R&D spending has skyrocketed and according to all forecasts, continues to grow at a remarkable rate. This, of course, translates into similar growth in grants to investigational sites.

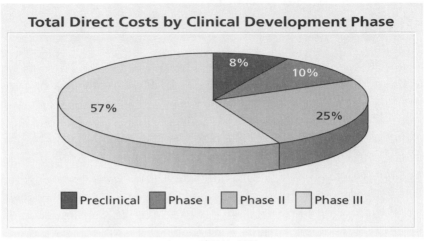

Total Direct Costs by Clinical Development Phase

8%
10%
57%
25%

■ Preclinical ■ Phase I □ Phase II □ Phase III

Source: PhRMA, 1999

In 1980, pharmaceutical and biotechnology companies that are members of Pharmaceutical Research and Manufacturers of America (PhRMA, the lobbying organization for the pharmaceutical industry) spent an estimated two billion dollars on research and development. In 1995, they poured $14.4 billion into R&D. Moreover, during the same period, the biotechnology industry matured. In 1995, biotech companies spent an estimated $8.5 billion on research. Together, PhRMA members and biotech companies spent $23 billion on R&D in 1995. That represents a tenfold increase in R&D spending in 15 years. This trend continues unabated and biotech companies continue to form and grow in huge numbers. Even though the majority of all biotech companies eventually fail, in most cases, they do contract for research and clinical trials prior to their demise. Whether the company succeeds or fails, however, the clinical investigators usually get paid.

The downturn in medical reimbursement in conjunction with the massive increase in R&D spending has led to a multi-billion dollar clinical trial industry that has developed primarily in the United States but is also growing significantly in other parts of the world. In 1992, industry grants to U.S. investigators totaled $1.9 billion. By 1996, total grants to U.S. investigators had risen to nearly $3 billion. Last year the figure approached $5 billion. In 1996, the average grant size was about $33,000. Since then, because of increased size and complexity of trials, it is likely that an average grant is closer to $45,000. There are well over 100,000 grants awarded yearly worldwide and 50,000 to 60,000 in the United States alone.

Of course, it is difficult to make judgments based on average gross revenues of grants. This is because the size and complexity of trials vary so greatly. Also, overall gross revenues do not translate into net in a clear manner. For example, it is not uncommon for payments in Alzheimer trials to exceed $10,000 per patient. However, these trials tend to be very labor intensive for the site, and there may be many costly procedures included that have to be paid for out of this budget. So, if a site entered 10 patients, at $10,000 each, this study would gross $100,000. But, if because of costly brain scans and the amount of labor required to conduct the trial, $9,000 is spent for each patient, then the site nets only $10,000 on this trial.

On the other hand, that site might contract to run a tension headache trial that requires only one brief visit and pays $500 per patient for 100 patients. It costs the site only $50 for each patient because there are no tests and minimal labor. Here the site nets $45,000 on a study that grosses half of the previously discussed Alzheimer trial.

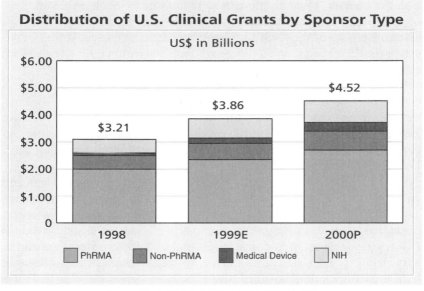

Source: CenterWatch Analysis, 2000, PhRMA; NIH

Who Gets the Grants?

Through the 1980s, clinical research was conducted primarily by physicians affiliated with academic medical institutions. Although there was some opportunity for the community physician to become involved, the pharmaceutical companies greatly preferred to work with physicians who could lend the prestige of an academic affiliation to their studies. Also, there wasn't a lot of choice because academic institutions were the only places that were familiar with the research process. Almost all other physicians had, at that time, no understanding of what participation in clinical trials required. More than 80% of all industry grants were, therefore, awarded to academic physicians.

This began to change in the 1980s. The emergence of managed care organizations put new economic pressures on pharmaceutical companies and physicians alike. Pharmaceutical companies, because of some real and perceived price controls on their products, had to convert themselves from relatively ineffective, low pressure industries to lean, competitive organizations. Time to market for new products became a major concern and cost of development a real but secondary issue. Physicians saw the beginning of a trend that still is in effect today: the reduction of their income and autonomy. The result of managed care was to make both pharmaceutical companies and the practicing medical community lean and hungry.

The obvious target for improving the development process was the clinical trial phase. Invariably clinical trials exceeded enrollment periods and over-ran budgets. Months and years were lost due to inefficiencies and lack of attention. The pharmaceutical companies were actually looked at with disdain by many of the academic researchers. It was almost as if the investigators condescended to accept huge grants. They would do the trials when they had the time.

The sponsoring companies began to look for more effective, quicker and cheaper ways to push their products through clinical trials. Many community physicians were looking for new cash flows into their practice. Academic physicians continued to produce poorly, not to pay attention to details, and to be inordinately expensive. Some institutions tacked on overhead charges as high as 60% of the entire budget.

The transition to highly motivated, independent investigators began and continues to gain steam even today. These individuals were highly responsive to the industry and much cheaper. Slowly and gradually, highly sophisticated, independent investigators began to grab market share. Instead of IRB approval taking two months, for example, it took two weeks. Instead of a trial requiring eight signatures and a slow lengthy review by an institution's legal department, one signature with no legal review resulted in instantaneous turnaround on contracts. Instead of a trial being delegated to the newest intern on the service, the actual investigator with whom the company contracted would be involved. Most important, patient enrollment improved dramatically. The private sector was beginning to pay attention to the trials.

By 1996, approximately 55% of industry grants for clinical research were awarded to investigators at academic medical centers. Slightly more than one third of the three billion dollars in grants awarded in 1996 went to community physicians. This trend has continued to the point where, today, over half of all grants are awarded to private researchers.

Academic institutions have attempted to stem the flow by developing offices for clinical research. The decrease in funding has been noticed, and many institutions have begun programs to market themselves and their investigators to the pharmaceutical community. Great intellectual capital remains at these institutions, and their efforts have had an impact. There seems to be a slowing of the bleeding, but these facilities have a long way to go to actually reverse the process. They remain inefficient, hampered by multiple layers of red tape and high overhead.

Private enterprise has responded to the huge potential represented by clinical trial grants. The number of independent sites and investigators has increased dramatically. In 1990, only 5,000 individual investigators were identified as filing 1572s. A 1572 is a form that must be signed by every principal investigator who does a trial in the United States. There will be more about this in a later chapter, and a 1572 is appended to this book. In 1996 there were almost 25,000 1572s filed. Today the number approaches 50,000. Obviously, both the number of clinical trials and the number of investigators who wish to do them are increasing.

The vacuum created by academia's inefficiency has become apparent to several varieties of entrepreneurs. These include those physicians who have developed dedicated research sites. There are several hundred of these sites scattered throughout the United States as well as some developing in Latin America and Europe. If run well, these are highly lucrative. Today, they are frequently sought for acquisition by developing SMOs. The average revenues for these dedicated sites have increased from $535,000 in 1993 to $1 million in 1996 and today exceed $1.5 million.

Site Management Organizations (SMOs)

SMOs have become increasingly visible over the last 10 years. Their strategies vary, but basically, they attempt to market a group of sites to the industry. They tout the advantages of contracting multiple sites through their one central organization. Standardization of sites, better and more consistent enrollment, and ease of developing one contract and one payment for multiple sites are but a few of the reasons suggested for why SMOs are a better way to go. To date, the SMOs have not adequately proved their claims, and, while being very visible, they have only captured about 3% of the market.

Sometimes SMOs will look outside their own sites and contract with practices and investigators in order to do clinical trials in specific medical areas or to find patients. The contracted investigator will supply the medical expertise and frequently will be asked to recruit patients from his or her own practice. The SMO will supply the study coordinator, the regulatory support and the trial. The contracted investigator will either work from his or her own office and the SMO will send its people there, or vice versa. This can frequently prove to be a good way for novice investigators to learn the business.

SMOs have been the darlings of Wall Street for many years even though initial public offerings have not done well. The first SMO to go public was Future Healthcare. This proved a disaster when fraudulent bookkeeping practices were revealed, and the upper management wound up being tried and convicted. A second public offering was done by Collaborative Clinical Research, and while no fraud was involved here, the company and its stock have done very poorly. Still, there was much interest in backing SMOs in the venture capital marketplace

Research Networks

In response to the increased competition for grants and the emergence of SMOs, many physicians engaged in clinical research on a part- or full-time basis have joined together to form research networks. A network may be general in scope or may focus on conducting research in one specific therapeutic area. Networks have formed that focus on ophthalmology, rheumatology, gastroenterology, oncology, neurology and other specialties.

The governing principles of the research network vary widely. Some are true consortiums owned largely by the investigators. Others involve loose affiliations among investigators banding together primarily for marketing purposes. In the first instance, each investigator member buys an ownership share in the network. The initial investment varies greatly, from a few thousand dollars to $25,000 or more. In return, the investigator expects that the network's management will secure grants and provide management expertise. It has been the goal of many of these networks to eventually do an initial public offering (IPO), but, to date, none have succeeded.

Depending on the structure of the network, the investigator may agree to work exclusively or nonexclusively for that network. In exclusive networks, all trials and grants must go through the network. This is fine if the network can keep a site busier than it would be without the network. Otherwise, it is probably a losing proposition for the site. In nonexclusive networks, the investigator is usually not required to accept a grant for any particular trial and may still secure trials on his or her own.

There are several benefits to joining an investigator-owned consortium. The network can provide many additional grants and trials. Its management expertise can facilitate contractual agreements and regulatory submissions. The network can even supply additional help in the form of part-time coordinators, if needed. And, if any of these networks realize their goal of going public, an investigator member could cash out.

More loosely affiliated networks usually provide fewer benefits but also fewer risks. First, these tend to cost less to join. Many of these networks simply hire one or two individuals to act as marketing and central administrative personnel. This type of arrangement has less potential to develop into a public offering, but currently, no network has gone public anyway.

As previously mentioned, there are potential downsides to network participation. A network is only as good as its worst investigator. If one of your associates performs poorly, or, worse, behaves in an unethical way, then this association has the potential to seriously damage your reputation. And in this industry, your reputation is your major asset. Another issue is the cost of membership. Some of these networks charge the participants up to 25% of a given contract. This fee can only be subtracted from the investigator grant because there is no budget item that the sponsor will pay to cover this charge. This is fine, if the network has the ability to negotiate a significantly higher budget for the site or can bring in enough work to cover their costs with something left over to give the site some additional profit.

There are multiple potential pathways for a novice investigator to explore clinical research. One would be through an SMO or a coordinator organization. Another might be involvement through your practice management organization. A network, if opened to inexperienced investigators, would also be a choice. And, if you have the desire and the perseverance, you could train yourself to participate in clinical research through some basic reading and "a little help from your friends," particularly if any of them are currently involved in clinical research. More about this in a later chapter.

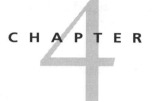

CHAPTER 4

The Players

- The Sponsors
- The Contract Research Organization (CRO)
- The Study Conduct Provider or Investigative Site
- The Patient and the Patient Advocate

This chapter will familiarize you with the different organizations that are involved in conducting clinical research. Each has a unique perspective and an important role in the development of new pharmaceutical products.

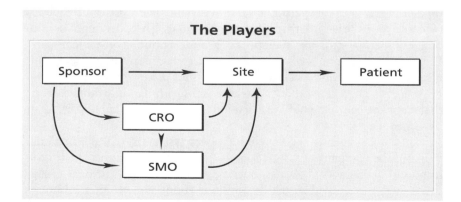

The Players

Sponsor → Site → Patient

Sponsor → CRO

CRO → SMO

Sponsor → SMO

SMO → Site

CRO/SMO → Site

The Sponsor

The pharmaceutical company, or sponsor, provides the drug itself and has the ability to structure and manage the overall process from the discovery period to the marketing of the drug.

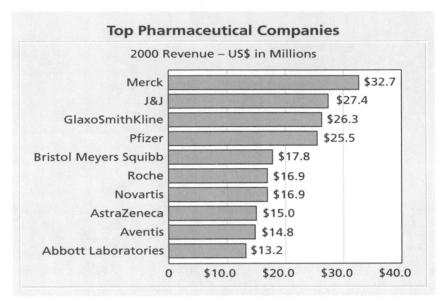

Top Pharmaceutical Companies

2000 Revenue – US$ in Millions

Company	Revenue
Merck	$32.7
J&J	$27.4
GlaxoSmithKline	$26.3
Pfizer	$25.5
Bristol Meyers Squibb	$17.8
Roche	$16.9
Novartis	$16.9
AstraZeneca	$15.0
Aventis	$14.8
Abbott Laboratories	$13.2

Source: PharmaBusiness, November 2000

There are different titles for individuals with whom you will interact at the sponsoring company, so be prepared to interchange the titles given here with others. One of the most important people you will interact with is the clinical research associate (CRA), also referred to as the field monitor or the regional clinical associate (RCA). This is the individual who visits your site periodically to collect data and monitor records for accuracy. In general, this is your connection to the company, and the relationship you and your coordinator create with this person is very important. The CRA can frequently promote your site as a participant in future studies. The CRA might be your best avenue for crossing therapeutic groups within a given company. Depending on a company's structure, a CRA may monitor all therapeutic areas or be therapeutic specific. If a CRA cannot place you into other studies, there is a good chance, if your relationship with that individual is poor, that he or she can veto your participation if you are recruited to participate by someone else.

The clinical scientist (CS) or clinical research scientist (CRS) is that individual at the company who functions as the in-house monitor. The CS collects and reviews data, issues queries and deals with adverse events. Frequently, this individual makes decisions about site selection. Although the sites' contact with the CS is generally less than with the CRA, it is important to get to know this individual, at least on the phone, and to interact in a positive fashion here as well. Sometimes, the CS and the CRA are the same individual.

The medical monitor (or medical expert or project team leader) is almost always a physician. This is usually the individual who is in charge of the entire protocol and is probably running several simultaneous protocols with the same drug. The medical monitor has the final say in determining which sites will be selected to participate in any given trial. Also, this individual is a resource for all medical questions involving the drug or the protocol. The relationship with the medical monitor is important and can be enhanced by the site's good performance. This is an individual that the site can make look really good or, conversely, look terrible to his or her superiors.

There are other important individuals to interact with at the sponsor company, such as the auditors and the contract manager, but they will interact less frequently with the site. The contract manager who is also known as the clinical administrator often negotiates the budget and cuts the grant checks. Again, names and titles will vary from company to company. It is important, however, for the investigator to understand the responsibility of all the individuals he or she deals with at the sponsoring company. This allows the investigator to interact more appropriately and also to solicit work in the future. Ask the CRA to draw you an organizational chart.

The Contract Research Organization (CRO)

Sponsoring companies can also choose how they want to implement their trial. Sometimes, either because their staff is fully occupied, or because a contract research organization (CRO) has specific expertise in a therapeutic or geographic area, the sponsoring company might choose to outsource some of the work. This work might include site selection and monitoring, medical writing and statistical analysis.

A CRO is defined, according to federal regulations, as an independent contractor that assumes one or more of the obligations of a sponsor, e.g., design of a protocol, selection monitoring of investigations, evaluation of reports, and preparation of materials to be submitted to the FDA.

Today there are approximately 1,000 active CROs worldwide. They range in size from massive companies such as Quintiles whose gross revenues exceed a billion dollars a year to small mom-and-pop shops that survive on a few hundred thousand in revenue. This industry is extremely tumultuous, and each year there are many failures and acquisitions.

The CRO industry grew up because it was more cost-effective for the pharmaceutical industry to use external companies during peak times of need rather than to hire staff whom they had to support during slow times as well. As time went on, the CROs became more and more experienced in the drug development process, and many pharmaceutical companies became less knowledgeable. A large CRO such as Covance or Quintiles, for example, might participate in the development of four or five drugs of a particular class for the same indication, while a sponsor would likely participate in only one.

CROs are very diverse in nature and structure, and many specialize in specific industry niches. Some do only data management while others do just FDA submissions. Some specialize in specific therapeutic arenas, and, if your practice concentrates on the same area, then a good connection with that particular CRO might give you the opportunity to participate in a lot of trials.

The majority of CROs are involved with the identification of investigators and the conduct of clinical trials. In today's highly competitive market, these companies compete on many fronts, including their ability to identify the best, most productive sites. And, truthfully, because CROs concentrate on this component of the business, they frequently have a high level of sophistication. They generally have databases of sites, do feasibility studies, and generally approach utilization better than sponsors do. I say "generally" because there is a wide variation in the levels of experience and knowledge across CROs and, frequently, within the same CRO.

Because of the accelerated growth of CROs, many of their employees are young, inexperienced individuals who are drafted into the industry right out of college. So when you, as a novice investigator, deal with one of these organizations, you might find someone with even less experience on the other side of the table.

Another interesting issue regarding CROs is that opportunity for advancement for employees at a given organization pyramids rather steeply. This means that the only chance for self-advancement for many of the people you come to know at one organization requires them to change companies. I call this phenomenon the "guppy syndrome." This means that a site with a good reputation at one company soon finds itself with business from two companies. The same, by the way, applies to less-than-stellar performers.

There has been much concern, in the clinical investigator community, that CROs frequently usurp a portion of an investigator's grant and use it to make their own company more profitable at the site's expense. I believe that this happens only rarely. Usually, and even when a grant is administered by the CRO, it is a separate line item and is accounted for from a separate pool. Actually, it is quite dangerous for a CRO to act in this fashion because if the trial does not go as well as expected, then the sponsor will immediately assume that it was because of this type of financial misconduct. The CRO could lose a contract worth millions and could destroy a relationship that could bring in millions more. By the way, a good profit margin for a CRO might be 16%, much lower than what is possible at the site level.

CROs can introduce you to the industry. If you perform well in a specific area, they are likely to have additional drugs to test in that area in the not too distant future. And, if you perform well in one therapeutic area, they are more likely to give you a chance to work in others. You see, in general, project people who work for CROs go from therapeutic area to therapeutic area themselves. It is likely that they will take a good investigator along for the ride or at least refer him or her to their coworkers.

There are multiple guides and lists of CROs available. One is published by CenterWatch, and another is a product of the Drug Information Association. It is likely that there are several CROs in close geographic proximity to you right now. A call to these organizations is a good way to begin to solicit trials.

Recently, some of the larger CROs have begun to create preferred investigator networks. As long as these networks do not require exclusivity from the investigators, they are beneficial to the site. In general, the purpose of these networks is to create a prioritized relationship for the CRO at extremely productive sites. This enables the CRO to utilize these relationships in marketing and conduct of their trials, thereby giving them an edge over the competition. The benefit for the site is, of course, to keep them as busy as possible.

The individuals with whom you interact at the CRO are very similar in title and background to those with whom you would interact at the sponsoring companies. Again, make sure you understand the organization for which you are working. Ask for organizational charts and keep them on file. Include telephone numbers and titles. These will be of value when you look for future trials.

CROs are good partners when you are first getting your feet wet in clinical trials. They are also a necessary partner as you create a clinical trials business because today, a large and growing percentage of clinical trials come through these organizations. A CRO is more likely to guide you through the trial process if you are new. It is simply because it is their business to make trials work. Sponsors are worried about many other things. Ultimately, though, experienced investigators prefer to deal directly with sponsors because it is simpler. There are fewer chefs making the soup, and the relationships you build with sponsors translate more easily into papers, additional trials with the same compound, and permanence.

The Study Conduct Provider or Investigative Site

The Medical Institution and Integrated Health Care System
As other potentially lucrative cash streams have dried up, more and more medical institutions and integrated health systems have begun to become more involved in clinical research. Fifteen years ago, almost all research was accomplished in academic centers. These centers have continually lost industry-sponsored research. This is because they had considered this research their due and in the past, they did nothing to accommodate or facilitate the trials. This has changed. Many universities are now paying attention

to industry sponsored trials and trying very hard to lure them back. A common approach is to develop a central office that contracts and manages trials, distributing the work to members of the staff. Also, this central agency deals with regulatory affairs, lends assistance to the investigator, and takes a substantial cut of the revenue for the university.

This approach has only been moderately effective. While some problems have been solved, others are embedded in the academic environment and extremely difficult to alter. Facilitation of trials might require a cultural change that is just too distant from the current situation to ever achieve. Nevertheless, several major academic institutions, including Duke University, University of Rochester and Columbia Presbyterian, have established aggressive and effective CRO services as part of their clinical research development.

Integrated health care systems seem to be nimbler than academic centers, but, for the most part, have not been able to facilitate clinical research. This is probably because it is still a fairly minor cash stream compared to all the other potentials. Also, these systems seem inundated with so many other issues and problems, clinical trials just have not claimed an important position. In the few cases it has, the approach has been less astute and informed than you would expect.

Integrated systems bring a lot of potential to the trial process, and it is likely that they will continue to dabble in this arena. Eventually, one of these systems will get it right and capture a significant portion of the market.

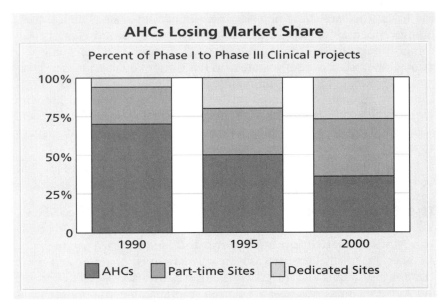

Source: CenterWatch

The Part-Time Investigator

This is the way most investigators begin doing clinical research. Most investigators incorporate clinical research into their practice by attempting involvement in one trial. This is a relatively risk-free way to test the water. There is a standing pool of subjects, patients in the practice, who are already predisposed to participate because of their ongoing relationship with the physician.

This is the model that is explored, for the most part, in this book. There are multiple issues as a physician moves to incorporate research into his or her practice, but as this happens, the practice should improve, not suffer. To do this properly requires that a balance be maintained between time spent practicing medicine and doing clinical research.

How Investigator Stipends Can Translate Elsewhere

When I was involved in the placement of a trial requiring "virgin congestive heart failure" patients it was suggested that we go to a site in Estonia to take advantage of the lack of available treatment for this disorder in that country, thereby making it easier to find patients for this pivotal trial. After identifying a site and interacting with a very enthusiastic investigator, I decided to make a site visit myself.

My initial impression of the site was negative because the office was small and cramped and the patient volume seemed overwhelming. While I waited to see the investigator, I counted 23 patients in the waiting room. This already seemed like an inordinate burden to a solo cardiologist and his obviously harried staff.

However, after I interviewed the investigator, I was very impressed by his knowledge, experience and enthusiasm for the project. Finding myself in a quandary, I asked him how he intended to handle the intense schedule of events, which require daily visits for each subject over a three-week period. He responded that he intended to schedule all 12 patients over the same three-week period and to close his office to anyone else except emergency patients. Then, after the trial he planned a two-week paid vacation for himself and his entire staff. Apparently, the stipend we offered for this trial compared favorably with his entire earnings for the previous year.

By the way, he did a great job.

Physicians who participate in research while maintaining their practice are those who are most frequently sought to participate in clinical trials and research by sponsors and CROs alike. It is here, in this setting, that the industry is most comfortable in placing its trials. Also, it is here where clinical trials have the greatest potential to transform the physicians into prescribing assets once the product is approved.

A physician does not have to be a "thought leader" to participate in trials. First of all, most thought leaders are not productive in this setting. Also, it is frequently difficult for the employees at the CROs and pharmaceutical companies to approach and interact with the thought leaders. Actually, placing things in perspective, thought leaders in general are less important than they used to be in the marketing of new products. Most practicing physicians understand that these highly respected individuals are frequently sponsored by the sponsor whose product they represent. This immediately discounts what they say. Also, we, as practicing physicians in this modern age of information, have access to multiple thought leaders, making the opinion of any one less significant. In fact, if we were to take this line of reasoning one step further, physicians are themselves less important in determining their own prescribing habits. Today pharmaceutical companies circumvent the entire medical establishment and market directly to the consumer.

Again, if clinical research is introduced into a practice in a way that neither threatens staff nor patients, the effects should enhance the growth of a practice. The perception that you or your group of physicians are on the cutting edge of medicine, continue to grow and educate yourself, and are endorsed by large pharmaceutical companies will only add to your practice's prestige. This is to say nothing of what becoming a lecturer and author of medical articles will do.

Many of the same forces that are driving American physicians to look carefully at clinical research are also applicable to the medical communities outside the United States. As previously stated, SMOs are developing in all corners of the world, and the FDA is more commonly reviewing and allowing foreign data in the NDA (new drug application). It is not uncommon for

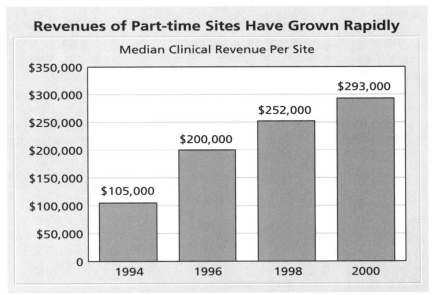

Source: CenterWatch

sponsoring companies to perceive future marketing advantages by doing some of the trials outside the United States. Also, it is not uncommon for a sponsor to place a trial outside the United States because the FDA has created some regulatory hurdles in the United States that can be circumvented by placing the study in Europe or South America. Sometimes, with certain indications, it is simply easier to find patients in other countries. For example, there is an extraordinarily high rate of hepatitis in China.

The major problem with conducting trials outside of the United States is that quality can be poor. Most sites in other parts of the world do not have a good understanding of Good Clinical Practices. And even if they did, they might not pay much attention to them. The FDA is one of the few regulatory bodies with any teeth at all patrolling the research industry. An investigator in Europe can actually fabricate a patient in a clinical trial, be discovered and suffer no serious consequences.

This is not, however, just an enforcement issue. There are also cultural and language differences that make the medical communities in other parts of the world less likely to adhere to a protocol, particularly if that protocol is designed for conduct by American physicians and based on standard treatment in the United States.

Despite all these issues, slowly and surely, harmonization is occurring. Eventually, like all other industries, American investigators will have to compete on a global basis.

The Dedicated Site

A dedicated site is a research center that does only clinical research. There is no practice of any other type carried out at this location. These sites are usu-

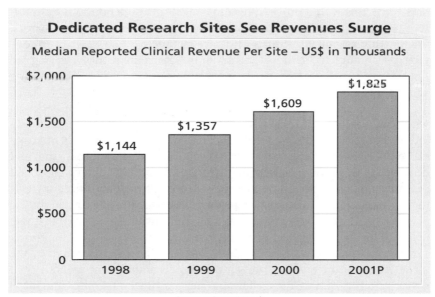

Dedicated Research Sites See Revenues Surge

Median Reported Clinical Revenue Per Site – US$ in Thousands

Source: CenterWatch

ally run by a physician or a physician in association with a business partner, both of whom usually dedicate their full time and attention to this venture. There are several hundred dedicated sites across the United States, and they seem to be the most consistent and productive segment of the investigator industry. These sites are capable of producing five million dollars a year in revenue or even, in a few cases, more. They are normally the pampered child of an entrepreneurial physician who has developed a highly efficient and productive organization. These sites are highly profitable. It is not unusual for the physician running a site like this to take home income in the area of seven figures. Such sites can employ 30 to 100 full-time people and run up to 100 trials a year. These sites frequently depend on sophisticated recruiting mechanisms to fill their trials. They may have several individuals whose only job is recruitment and an extensive computerized telephone system running 18 hours a day, simply for the purpose of soliciting patients and building a patient database.

These sites usually require years to build and live on their reputations. It has recently become somewhat more difficult to establish new centers like this because the industry has grown so much in the recent past. Consequently, it is harder to establish a large enough reputation to fuel an operation of this dimension.

On occasion, you will hear these sites referred to as "study mills," a rather disparaging term that seems to imply that these sites only consider the commercial side of the business. Certainly there is less camouflage of the importance of the dollar at these sites, but those individuals who run these clinics seem, for the most part, to maintain a high level of enthusiasm for the science as well. No question though, these are finely tuned businesses. If you know of such a site in your area and can wangle the chance to spend a few days there, this would prove to be an excellent introduction to the clinical research arena. It also would be an excellent place to train your coordinators.

Recently, several individuals who have run these centers have been convicted of fraudulent behavior, and several of them are actually serving jail time. This type of thing has made some sponsors more leery of employing such sites to conduct trials.

Finally, because these sites are not associated with practicing physicians who prescribe, they are seldom sought to participate in late-stage trials. The lack of association with a practice can make certain types of trials impossible to do. For example, it would be difficult to do a "strep throat" trial at a dedicated site because enrollment depends upon the ability to solicit patients to join the trial when they appear at the physician's office for treatment. The same would be true for patients requiring hospitalization during or as part of the trial. These sites could not be considered in a trial that was designed for "post-operative pain post-hysterectomy."

In conclusion, dedicated sites are generally the most productive, the most clearly commercial and probably the gold standard for productivity in a wide variety of clinical research trials. They are, however, limited and inappropriate for other trials.

The Site Network

Site networks are either formal or informal associations of investigators, usually established for the purpose of promoting work for all members. As sites grow and develop, a major issue is always the pipeline. As more and more individuals are hired to service this segment of the practice, more trials are required to keep them busy and the busier they are, the more profitable the enterprise becomes. This is because there are some basic fixed costs that you encounter whether you do one or two trials, or 15 or 20 trials. Once these costs are covered, this business becomes increasingly profitable. The point to focus on here is that the volume of trials is directly proportional to profitability.

Some of these site network organizations hire a small group of marketing personnel and a small administrative staff to collect dues and help them jointly contract and recruit. Other networks are as simple as telephone trees amongst friends. I believe many of these are quite effective. There is, however, some downside to these associations. This is the same as with SMOs and hybrids which are discussed later in this chapter. Any network, association or group is only as good as its weakest link. Even if your site does a great job, if one of your associates does poorly, then your site will be tarred with the same brush. There is an old axiom in marketing circles that one negative experience requires 12 positive experiences to cancel it out. I think that this ratio is a correct one when applied to clinical research as well

The Site Management Organization (SMO)

Site management organizations are an interesting, but not new, phenomenon. These organizations have been created by entrepreneurial spirits who believe that there are better ways to do trials than the traditional, individual sites functioning under a physician director or the academic centers. SMOs are enterprises that attempt to bring business principles to the "mom-and-pop" realm of investigators.

SMOs attempt to standardize and string together a series of sites. They usually introduce the same approach at each site, so that, they claim, the quality of work is better standardized. They utilize centralized marketing and recruiting strategies to attract both trials and patients to fill those trials. SMOs claim that they are a better "mousetrap," but there is little proof that this is so. While there are some notable successes in a few scattered trials, there have been no substantiated trends that would verify this.

There are several different SMO models. Some SMOs have been formed by stringing together a group of well-established research sites. The site is purchased utilizing a combination of cash, stock and future options. Another method is to establish or "green field" new sites. These obviously require more work to establish and take a while to come up to speed, but, of course, are much cheaper to acquire.

Some SMOs do not establish free-standing, independent sites but look to create partnerships with practicing physicians. These organizations create a research potential in large, ongoing practices. They install research coordinators, equipment, managers and all the other necessities into these sites. This is an attractive model because it usually costs less to establish and has a built-in patient base.

Recently SMOs have begun to develop outside the United States. There are currently several established SMOs in the United Kingdom. There is some additional rationale for the development of these organizations there because it is frequently impossible to recruit patients into trials without the participation of the specific generalists to which each patient is assigned. The system in the Netherlands is slightly less restrictive, so the SMOs established there actually use independent dedicated structures as the base for their organization. Area physicians refer patients to them for a fee. In France, dedicated sites are being created. These sites hire area doctors equipped with their patient rolls and who function as investigators, assisted by the full-time staff at these facilities.

There have already been a few SMOs that have gone public. Indeed, it seems that most of them have been created with a strategy of eventually doing the same. To date, however, none that have gone public has been successful. The problem is that these organizations are being built, in general, to be sold, not to be profitable. Consequently there seems to be diminished interest by venture capitalists and the other powers that be on Wall Street.

It can be safely stated, at this point in time, that SMOs have not proved to be successful ventures. Although there are multiple models in existence, none have been productive to the extent required to ensure ongoing viability.

There are many reasons for this. When SMOs contract for clinical trials, they almost never receive additional payment. On the contrary, SMOs frequently negotiate prices down in the hopes that this will induce a sponsoring company to utilize more of the SMO's sites. In general, the support of an SMO's superstructure requires 25% of the gross revenues of a study. If one considers that most studies provide a profit margin of between 25% and 50%, it become clear that SMOs are at a decided disadvantage in competing against nonaffiliated sites and also might have difficulty remaining profitable at all.

Frequently, SMOs will state that, as their organizations grow, overhead is spread among more sites and, therefore, the percentage decreases. This would be true if the overhead didn't rise along with the growth of the organization. Unfortunately, there will be some corresponding increase in the cost of maintaining the superstructure. Also, it is incredibly difficult to keep all sites functioning at full capacity all the time. Pipeline becomes an overwhelming issue as these organizations grow.

A second problem is intrinsic to the personalities of most good investigators. These individuals tend to work best for themselves, and it can be difficult to inspire their total participation when entrepreneurial motivations are removed or diminished.

SMOs, to date, have not proven their ability to recruit patients faster while presenting cleaner data. There have been a couple of studies where this has occurred, but no consistent pattern has emerged.

It is entirely possible that SMOs are selling a product to an industry that has little positive impetus to adopt it, while, at the same time, there are several reasons not to go ahead.

These negative reasons include the fact that the inclusion of an SMO into a trial adds another hierarchy to deal with. If a company is already utilizing a CRO, then the CRO and the SMO begin to replicate each other's function thereby confusing reporting issues, IRB issues, emergency procedures and pretty much all other aspects of dealing with the site. The net effect of redundant superstructures can easily translate into a loss of productivity.

Another negative incentive, from the sponsor and CRO's perspective, involves the questionable wisdom of empowering the investigators in general. Why would one want to deal with a unionized site if there is no need for it? Sites are simply easier to control, replace and otherwise manipulate if they are dealt with on an individual and competing basis. It is unlikely than any one site alone will place a large multi-center trial in jeopardy. Three or five sites might.

Another issue is that most therapeutic groups developing drugs like and need to develop strong, personal relationships with investigators in their arena, some of which extend back to medical school and residency training. They bring with them an element of comfort and trust that will totally stifle an SMO's attempt to intercede. Generally, by the way, these are the investigators who are used over and over again. Clearly, they would not be subject to displacement by an SMO. The relationship involving the placement of clinical trials is the primary one.

The Hybrid

Another format that has recently emerged is the hybrid. This is an organization that functions as a CRO but also owns sites, thereby combining the SMO and CRO concept into one. Those who run these organizations claim that they function better because the working paradigm is established and runs better than a system that requires multiple interfaces. Usually, these hybrids specialize in one or two therapeutic areas. They also sell their services as either a CRO or an SMO.

These organizations are perceived as competitors by the CRO industry, consequently, they cannot look to CROs to give them any work. This decreases their customer base tremendously. Also, part of the job of the CRO is to monitor the conduct of the trial at the site level. If the site and the CRO are part of the same company, does this decrease the objectivity of the monitor? How many companies would diminish their own reputation by reporting either errors of omission or commission at their own company?

To date, these companies have experienced some tough sledding, but many of the people running them are quite experienced and determined to make this model successful.

The Practice Management Organization

Like integrated systems and universities, practice management organizations are attempting to make inroads into clinical research. These companies believe that they can introduce research to the practices that they manage or own and create a new cash stream into that practice. The idea is good, but so far the execution has not been. Currently, none of these organizations have been successful in this endeavor. These organizations have essentially created captive SMOs, and in so doing, have repeated most of the mistakes made by those companies. They have been top-heavy and cumbersome. They have complicated the process of doing trials for the sponsors and CROs as opposed to simplifying and facilitating. Also, they have missed an essential element of the puzzle in that not all physicians will be able to or are interested in doing clinical trials. Good investigators usually identify themselves through their active pursuit of and interest in the area. This is not something that can be foisted upon practices.

Currently, practice management organizations seem to be fighting for their existence on many fronts, and it is likely that they have more pressing issues and larger fish to fry at the current time. It seems unlikely that there will be a concerted effort for involvement in clinical trials from this direction in the near future.

The Managed Care Organization

Managed care organizations can be divided into for-profit and nonprofit organizations. Today, all the growth is in the for-profit group. For-profit HMOs account for over 80% of the field and are fast gobbling up the non-profit group. This has significant impact on the conduct of clinical trials in managed care because it is actually possible to conduct some trials in non-profit organizations, provided the trials meet the criteria established by these organizations. In general, if sponsors want to do trials in managed care, the trials must address issues that are of importance to the HMO. But, with the right trial, nonprofit HMOs such as Kaiser can do an excellent job.

For-profit HMOs, on the other hand, have almost no interest in conducting clinical research. Clinical research merely interferes with the conduct of their business. There is no comfortable place to incorporate it into their system, and the fees paid are generally not enough to cause these massive organizations to want to change from business as usual.

For-profit HMOs are also not interested in subsidizing industry-sponsored research. This means that as long as the trials don't cost these companies money, they will cast a blind eye to their enrollees' participation in research. The problem occurs when you encounter the "zone of uncertainty." It is here, where there is a question of who is responsible for costs, where conflicts may occur.

It is common for most practicing physicians to fill trials with patients for whom they are capitated by HMOs. Except for rare instances, there are no problems in doing so. After all, the participation of a patient in a research protocol is a decision made between that patient and his doctor. This is not available for review by the insurance carrier, nor should it be. Incidentally, many physician-investigators believe that the only way they can make a profit from their capitated populations is to place these patients into clinical trials.

The Coordinator Organization

Coordinator organizations are actually a type of SMO. These are generally run by one or a group of experienced coordinators who have decided to set up an independent business. These function by enlisting area physicians as investigators. They place experienced coordinators into the physician's office and conduct the trial from there. They pay the physician a fee to cover his or her work as an investigator, and sometimes they pay additional rent and service charges to the practice. These coordinators generally acquire the trial, interface with the sponsor or CRO, do the regulatory work, and deal with all aspects of the trial, utilizing the physician for his or her patient base and medical expertise. The physician functions as the investigator and must see the patients when required to by the protocol, go to the investigator meeting, and sign off on the case report forms, in addition to other routine and normal investigator functions.

Actually, this is not a bad way to introduce yourself to research. The problem is that the physician remains dependent upon the coordinator organization for expertise in conducting the trial as well as for contacts to obtain the work. The physician earns at a better level than he or she would if the same amount of time was applied to his or her normal practice, however, the site and the investigator never mature. Of course, the majority of the payment is earned by the coordinators and not the site.

So, while this might be an acceptable solution for the short-term, it stifles the investigator and the site in the intermediate and long-run. The site never acquires the knowledge and connections to grow an independent, lucrative business.

The Patient and the Patient Advocate

The Institutional Review Board (IRB)

The institutional review board plays a central role in the drug approval process in the United States. These boards are generally created and run by hospitals or academic institutions. Over the last 10 years, however, commercial, or free-standing independent IRBs have made their way on to the scene. The composition of an IRB is determined by federal regulations and must include minority representation, scientific representation, moral representation and at least one individual who is not associated with the institution who is sponsoring the board. There must be at least five members, and members can be, and most frequently are, reimbursed for their time reviewing protocols and sitting in committee. It is the job of the IRB to review the moral and scientific ramifications of a given protocol. The board's first concern is for the safety and welfare of the subjects entering the trial.

The IRB will spend a good amount of time reviewing the protocol to ensure that the subjects are not placed in unnecessary danger or exposed to unnecessary risk. The IRB will also make a judgement whether the protocol is worth doing. But, the majority of the time spent by the IRB is devoted to review of the consent form. This is the form designed by the investigator (frequently with much help from the sponsor) that informs the patient of the procedures and dangers to which he or she exposes himself or herself when participating in the trial. There will be more about the creation and design of this form as well as the appropriate way to get "consent" in chapter nine. Also, there is a sample form appended to the book. Suffice it to say at this moment, that the consent form is required to cover specific points of information, to be written in language a sixth grader can comprehend, and to not mislead the patient in any way.

Not only must an investigator receive approval from a properly structured IRB prior to beginning a trial, the IRB must be periodically updated on the progress of the trial. Also, any change or amendments to the protocol must be approved by the IRB before they are put into operation. The IRB must be notified immediately of any serious, adverse events that occur either at your site or at any other site conducting the trial. So, you can see that the involvement of the IRB in a clinical trial is essential and ongoing.

IRBs charge for their services. The usual fees range from $1,500 to $2,500. There are frequently additional fees for amendment approvals and other actions. Although a sponsor or CRO will always reimburse a site for these fees, it's important to remember to include them in the budget. It is also important to note that an IRB does not have the right to review the investigator's contract with the sponsor. The investigator's fees and payment arrangements are private and should never be sent to the IRB

Obtaining IRB approval is frequently a bottleneck in the process, particularly when academic institutions are involved. And, if a trial is conducted on the physical grounds of an institution, or in any facility owned by a particular institution, that institution's IRB has jurisdiction and must be used as the IRB regarding that protocol, unless the institution waives its rights. This has tremendous potential to slow down the process because some IRBs meet monthly or even less frequently. Also, they may have very full schedules and there might be a waiting list for several months.

Frequent delays and hold-ups in the process have led to the development of commercial IRBs. These are businesses that contract with investigators to assume all the responsibilities of an IRB but do so in a very professional, effective manner. Normally, these IRBs meet weekly and allow an investigator to turn the approval process around in two weeks or less. These commercial IRBs enable sites to get a running jump on initiating the protocol. Remember, however, that these can only be utilized by sites that are not under the jurisdiction of their own institution's IRB. There are many commercial IRBs, including:

- **Chesapeake Research Review**
  The Chesapeake Building
  9017 Red Branch Road, Suite 100
  Columbia, Maryland 21045
  (410) 884-2900

- **Copernicus Group Institutional Review Board**
  118 MacKenan Drive, Suite 400
  Apex, NC 27511
  (888) 303-2224

- **New England Institutional Review Board**
  40 Washington Street, Suite 130
  Wellesley, MA 02481
  (781) 431-7577

- **Quorum Institutional Review Board**
  509 Olive Way, Suite 500
  Seattle, WA 98101
  (206) 448-4082

- **Shulman & Associates Institutional Review Board**
  760 Montgomery Road, Suite B
  Cincinnati, OH 45236
  (513) 792-9556

- **Western Institutional Review Board**
  3535 7th Avenue SW
  Olympia, WA 98502-5010
  (360) 943-1410

Sometimes CROs and sponsors use commercial IRBs as "central" IRBs. This means that the sponsoring company contracts with a specific IRB and requests that all sites participating in the trial submit their documents to this designated IRB. Again, if a site functions under an institution that has its own IRB, it may not be able to comply. Frankly, however, those sites that are free to utilize central IRBs have a leg up on others because this type of scenario can facilitate the process of a trial. A contract with a central IRB allows a company to submit all sites en masse and to get all of them approved at once. This is much easier than dealing with 15 separate IRBs, each with its own specific requirements. Also, it is easier to keep one IRB updated on serious adverse events and other issues. Finally, it's cheaper. Normally, a commercial IRB will give the sponsoring company a very hefty price break, if it submits more than one site at one time.

Each IRB has its own particular requirements and quirks. Whether you use a specific institution's IRB or a commercial IRB, it is important that you learn the requirements so there will be no unnecessary roadblocks in the approval process. Learn the specifics about how they want consent forms designed, protocols and amendments submitted and all other issues. Also, expect a visit from the IRB to your facility at some time. They are required to do so.

It is important to develop a good relationship with a specific IRB because the research process will work much better if you and the board move hand in hand.

The Patient

The patient makes the final decision regarding his or her participation. The reasons why people consider participation are many, but do not discount altruism as a major one. Many people simply want to help, particularly if they have been dealing with a chronic disease themselves. They want to improve their own condition, but there is also great concern for others who deal with the same disorder.

Sometimes the patient simply wants to please a doctor or nurse. You must be careful not to take advantage, as an investigator, in this scenario. One of the greatest motivations does remain the relationship between the patient and the study coordinator. These individuals often develop close attachments to each other as the trial proceeds.

Sometimes the stipends are the key. Even though the size of the payments to the patients are limited, during the course of a long study, payments can amount to significant dollars, particularly if you add the free medical treatment and free medications. It is sad but true that this is the only way some people can afford medical treatment.

Another important motivating factor is that clinical trial patients can obtain innovative and exciting drugs years before the drugs come to the market. This is of great significance when dealing with serious and life-threatening illnesses. Many times, when a trial of an innovative product proves efficacious, there are extensions of the trial created so subjects can be maintained on the therapy. Sometimes this is not possible, and patients find themselves waiting for the next trial with that product or the release of the drug to the market.

It is obvious that trials cannot be conducted without the good will and cooperation of patients. These individuals need, therefore, to be cared for and appreciated as they go through the process. Having participated in many trials as a subject, I know that the successful completion of a trial depends on the active commitment of both site personnel and subjects.

The Patient Recruitment Firm

It is not unusual for sponsoring companies or for CROs to hire a patient recruitment company to market clinical trials to the public. This is done to facilitate enrollment into these trials. Often recruitment firms charge millions of dollars for their services and utilize all mass media forums available, including newspapers, television, radio and the Internet. In fact, many of these companies are or have been acquired by large CROs.

The reason these companies are hired is because large, important (pivotal) trials often fall behind in enrollment. And, every day of delay in approval of an important product can cost that company between one and five million dollars. Again, these companies are hired by the sponsors, not the site.

These companies can make some portions of the investigators' job easier. If the firm is experienced and has done its job properly, they can inundate a site with potential candidates for a clinical trial. This is the advantage and also the disadvantage of working with them for the site. If a site does not carefully consider how many patients it can accommodate up front, that site might find itself spinning its wheels and inappropriately allocating time and resources, not only in this specific trial, but also in all its other trials and even in its routine non-research business.

Generally, these companies use a central clearing station. All subjects who respond to their advertisements are collected at this station and then distributed out to investigators in the patients' proximity. Depending on the contract, a varying amount of phone screening will be done. This means that, depending upon the telephone scripts, the referral to the site might be more or less valuable.

Before accepting referrals from a recruitment company, the investigator must allocate specific blocks of patient time to receiving and seeing the referred subjects. Herein lies the rub. If a site allocates too much time, then it uses its resources unproductively. If it allocates too little time, it wastes potential patients. Add the complicating factor that, many times, those patients referred from these services do not show up at all and the challenge of staffing appropriately becomes enormous.

So, if you agree to work in conjunction with these companies, it is important that you take it slowly at first. You must develop a feel for how many patients actually show up and how long it takes to conduct an initial visit with these new patients. After all, it is not as if you know these people as you do your own patients. A suggestion might be to allocate two patient slots initially, but to schedule three patients, or one and a half patients to each slot, until experience dictates further adjustments.

If a recruitment firm is involved in the trial and its services are offered to your site, you must seriously consider using it. Enrollment into clinical trials is always competitive. Your site will be compared to all others, and it is in your interest to be one of the top producers. This is one of the keys to bringing sponsors back over and over again. In fact, if a paper is produced at the end of the trial, the authors, usually all investigators, are most often listed in order of their productivity.

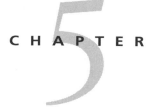

CHAPTER 5

Catch-22: How do You Secure Your First Grant?

- How to Gain Experience
- How to Get the Trial
- The Initial Site Visit

As you might expect, securing the first grant is the most difficult step to take. Once you have successfully conducted one trial, it becomes easier to obtain a grant for a second and third trial. But until you have that initial "experience" on your curriculum vitae (CV), you may find yourself caught in a Catch-22. Sponsors will want to know that you have conducted research before, and of course, you can't get that experience unless someone gives you that first grant.

There are ways, however, to surmount this hurdle. Remember, each year more than 5,000 physicians secure their first grants. The key is to follow a systematic strategy for breaking into this business.

How to Gain Experience

There are many ways to get research experience on your CV. Options range from functioning as a sub-investigator to an active investigator in your region, to contracting with an SMO. Scenarios vary, depending on whom you deal with, the type of study and what each party agrees to bring to the table. In this chapter, I will discuss several typical scenarios.

If you are connected with an academic institution or integrated health care system that has developed an active clinical research program, then this might be the best place to start. Many academic institutions have central research offices that contract with sponsoring companies while identifying investigators and assisting them in conducting the trial. Many of these central offices will offer the novice investigator an entire menu of study-related services to choose from, including providing the site with a trained coordinator. These services eat up most of the budget, but you have to remember that the goal here is to get started. You can worry about being profitable a little later. The same situation exists in many integrated health care systems, and there are even some practice management organizations that have begun to offer the same services.

Another way to develop some experience is to become a sub-investigator. If you have a friend or colleague who is actively involved as a researcher, you could spend some time in your colleague's office learning the ropes. As a sub-investigator, you can participate in the trial and not have to accept the full responsibilities of the principal investigator. Perhaps you could refer some of your patients into the trial. As long as your office was listed on the 1572, you could see study patients there. This is an excellent way to lay claim to some study experience and enhance your CV so that you will become attractive to the sponsors and CROs.

You can also gain research experience by signing an agreement with a coordinator's organization or an SMO that has you functioning as an investigator in your own office, utilizing your own patients and your own equipment. The organization with which you contract brings to your facility their coordinators and experience to make sure that the trial is conducted properly. Generally, the contract is between that organization and the sponsoring company or CRO. Consequently, they make the lion's share of the income, and the investigator is paid for his or her services. Actually, this is not a bad way to introduce yourself to research and to build your CV.

 ## The Workhorse

I was very impressed to be part of an elite and well-known group of investigators participating in a phase II trial of an innovative drug for hypertension. Out of the 10 investigators present, seven were famous for writing the papers and books the rest of us used to determine how we treat hypertension.

I told the medical monitor from the sponsoring company how flattered I was to be in such impressive company. He responded, "Don't be, we need you to actually do the work."

Another possible scenario is when a physician agrees to work in a freestanding site as contracted help. Instead of the organization coming to you,

you go to them. This is also a good way to get your feet wet, provided you can spare a consistent block of time from your daily activities. Be careful of restrictive covenants. The company you work for may try to restrict your participation in clinical research for several years, if you decide to go off on your own.

You should be able to locate a dedicated research site or an SMO in your area through contacts with the local medical community. You may also notice advertisements for study volunteers in the local paper or on the radio that have been placed by an SMO or dedicated research site. There is also a partial listing of SMOs and dedicated research sites on an internet site run by CenterWatch. The internet address is http://www.centerwatch.com. You can search for research centers by geographic location or therapeutic specialty.

If you are satisfied with the arrangement, it is fine to continue. However, after doing this a couple of times, you might want to try flying on your own. There are some things of which you need to be careful. First, when you sign an agreement with one of these companies, look for any restrictive covenant. If there is one and it extends beyond considerations for the specific trial on which you are working, you may not want to sign it. Don't accept general restrictions. A second consideration is the introduction of new individuals into your practice setting. These individuals can be disruptive, so make sure that you have worked out up front where they will work, with what they will be supplied, and other issues.

How to Get the Trial

Once you have the experience, there are many ways to find your first clinical trial. Below, I will discuss some proven ways, but for each one listed there probably exists many more not recorded here.

Talk to the Pharmaceutical Detail People

It is likely that every day a sales person from one of the pharmaceutical companies sits in your office. This individual can be a conduit into clinical research. First, drug companies know that physicians who are involved in clinical trials are more likely to prescribe that drug, once it is approved for market. Thus, detail people know that it is in their interest to get physicians involved in clinical research. It makes their job easier down the road. Furthermore, they know that if they can help a physician get started in research, the physician is likely to be more welcoming the next time they visit the office. Ask the detailers to provide you with the names, phone numbers and addresses of the people in their company who are directing research projects. If possible, get them to provide you with specific names for specific projects. Detailers may even be willing to set up meetings with project directors.

Frequently, detailers will be able to put you directly into phase IV post-approval trials, or even give you a grant, if you have a small research project you would like to design. The latter route is somewhat complex, but the former is an easy way to at least begin some research. Phase IV trials are actually becoming mandated more frequently by the FDA to serve as a long-term surveillance tool.

In general, these phase IV trials usually involve the completion of a few pages of case report forms for a small fee. It is not uncommon for the company to enlist several hundred to several thousand doctors to participate and for each to be asked to contribute five or 10 patients. This type of study is frequently a mechanism to introduce physicians to the new product, and these studies are run by the marketing division as opposed to the research division of the company that concentrates on phases I through III trials. Therefore, participation in phase IV does not frequently transfer into the separate research organization and that is the place you want to be. Still, if you do four or five late phase trials, you are likely to gain a little credibility. Most of the same principles and procedures apply. You will still probably be required to get IRB approval and to follow GCPs. The case report forms will be simple and the payments small, but it is a way to start. Do it and add the trial to your CV.

Write to the Pharmaceutical Companies

This is a time-honored way of breaking into the business. While the appendix includes a list of the top 10 pharmaceutical companies, also use the Physicians' Desk Reference or The Monthly Prescribing Reference to collect addresses and to develop lists of companies. You can have your coordinator call each company to identify research directors and therapeutic division leaders so you can specifically address your letters. Try and find the individuals who direct the research divisions, therapeutic areas and specific projects. Write a letter to each of them. Also, if the company keeps an investigator's databank, find out who runs that and request forms so you can have your site entered into it.

Your letter should include information about your specialty, board certification, patient demographics and any research experience you may have. You will want to include a copy of your CV. It should be signed, up-to-date and include any academic appointments you may have had. You will want to list any lectures, publications and society memberships as well. Make it look good.

In addition, the letter should detail what steps you have taken to prepare yourself and your site for clinical research. Mention any courses you have taken, specific changes you have made to your office, and talk a little about your coordinator. Make sure it is understood that he or she is completely dedicated to clinical research and not part-time. Also, particularly if your coordinator is experienced, include his or her CV along with your own. There is nothing that will attract more business than this simple step.

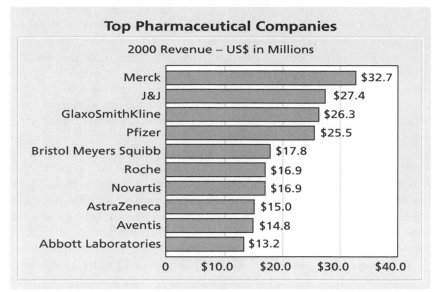

Top Pharmaceutical Companies

2000 Revenue – US$ in Millions

Company	Revenue
Merck	$32.7
J&J	$27.4
GlaxoSmithKline	$26.3
Pfizer	$25.5
Bristol Meyers Squibb	$17.8
Roche	$16.9
Novartis	$16.9
AstraZeneca	$15.0
Aventis	$14.8
Abbott Laboratories	$13.2

Source: PharmaBusiness, November 2000

Like all large organizations, pharmaceutical companies are not models of efficiency. A vast amount of time is wasted on deciding what studies to do and then on designing them. There is even more time wasted in operationalizing the trials. Consequently, by the time that they actually reach the investigators' hands, there is enormous pressure to move things along. However, it does not improve from this point forward. Over half the time a trial is started, the enrollment goals are not met.

There are many reasons why enrollment falls behind. The first is unrealistic expectations. Frequently those individuals designing trials are not, and never have been, practicing physicians. Often, therefore, the expectations of how easily a trial can be filled are not well-founded in experience. And, in most companies, there is not a good feasibility process in place. The assumptions are not reality-tested prior to becoming incorporated into the protocol.

Another problem is the inappropriate selection of investigators. The company may, for example, decide to place the study with many well-known thought leaders. While this ultimately will add a huge amount of intellectual capital and marketing potential to the mix, these doctors may be well removed from the patients about whom they currently write and teach. Also, the doctors might be so busy with other responsibilities that they have no time to actively participate.

Each pharmaceutical company has its own mechanism for the selections of sites to participate in clinical trials. And frequently, there are several different paradigms at the same company. An investigator cannot assume that any knowledge of his or her capabilities is necessarily transferable across different therapeutic teams or even within the same therapeutic area. The best way to ensure your selection as an investigative site is to continually build strong relationships up and down the line in the sponsoring organizations. For example, in some companies, the field monitors, who visit the sites, have a lot to say about which sites are selected for trials. In other companies, it is the clinical scientists or the medical monitors who make this choice. Sometimes marketing people are involved as well.

The bottom line here is that pharmaceutical companies look for sites that can quickly produce the promised number of patients with clean, reliable data. They want a site to be able to stand up to FDA inspections. If your site can do this, then it will be utilized over and over again.

Write to the CROs

CROs are involved in some component of over 50% of all clinical trials. CROs are frequently used by sponsors for site identification and selection. Also, some CROs do feasibility studies for the industry. In general, most CROs do have a more sophisticated approach to site identification. Almost all of them have internally developed investigator databases. It is, therefore, important to write the therapeutic groups at CROs, just like you would a sponsoring company, and it is also important to make sure you find the keeper of the database and get the proper forms sent to you so you can enter your site into it. At some CROs, there is a central and specific individual who does a lot of the site selection. Identify this person and you have accomplished a great deal.

Some CROs have feasibility groups that actively and continually query investigators about their ability to find patients to fill specific trials. In general, these groups go back to specific investigators who are part of the investigator database to supply information under confidentiality agreements. In many companies, the project teams who pick the investigators are disconnected from the feasibility group. However, sometimes a connection is maintained between the two and those investigators who donate their time in the feasibility process actually get the work in the trials.

The decision of whether the CRO or the pharmaceutical company chooses the investigator depends on the specific contract for a particular trial. It is a specified item and usually is contracted out when the sponsoring company is working in a new area or has exhausted its supply of investigators.

There are many sources of CRO lists. A list of the top CROs is included in the appendix. Another source is:

- **Drug Information Association (DIA)**
  501 Office Center Drive, Suite 450
  Fort Washington, PA 19034-3211
  (215) 628-2288

Tap Into Industry Publications and Databases

Several industry services can help novice investigators secure grants. There are many commercial databases that charge the site to place a listing. Then, these listings are distributed to the industry and the CROs at no charge. It is a good idea for a new investigative site to list itself in several of these because they are frequently used to identify sites. When placing your site information, it is a good idea to reach a little. List all those clinical areas where you think it might be possible for you to function effectively and list all types of trials where you feel you can participate. After all, you can always say no if approached about a trial you don't believe you can do. A good way to judge what constitutes an acceptable description of your site and capabilities is to look through the database or journal and look at what other sites have done. Then, model your advertisement accordingly. Usually it costs less than $100 to list your site in one of these publications and, of course, that money is rapidly recaptured with the acquisition of even one trial. Some of these listing services include:

■ **Research Investigator's Source, Inc.**
1500 Lilac Drive South, Suite 260
Minneapolis, MN 55416-1565
(800) 535-6365

■ **CenterWatch**
22 Thomson Place
Boston, MA 02210
(617) 856-5900

CenterWatch publishes a monthly newsletter that, in each issue, lists 20 to 30 pharmaceutical companies and CROs that are actively seeking investigators for upcoming trials. Investigators can use this information to apply for grants in their therapeutic areas. The annual cost of subscribing to the newsletter is $395.

CenterWatch also publishes an industry directory that lists, along with sponsors and CROs, investigative sites by geographic area and therapeutic area expertise.

Advertising in Industry Journals
Another approach is to promote your site in some of the journals commonly read in the pharmaceutical industry. A well-constructed ad placed in CenterWatch, Applied Clinical Trials, ACRP's The Monitor or the journal of the DIA can frequently yield results. It is probably better to construct an ad that is low key but gives those looking for sites enough information to follow up. Things that you will want to include are what types of trials you are interested in, the phase of work you would like to participate within, your staffing and experience and anything that would make you a uniquely effective site. Obtain a few back issues of each of these journals and then construct an ad that would seem to fit the model.

Long-Term Marketing Strategies
The best marketing any site can do, of course, is to perform well for sponsors and CROs. A site that starts studies quickly, fulfills contractual obliga-

tions regarding patient enrollment, and produces clean data will quickly find that it can grow through reputation alone. Sponsors and CROs will regularly return to the sites that meet these standards.

The Ice Man Cometh

During the site visit, it is important to demonstrate that you have read the protocol and have thought about how you will comply with the tiniest details. For example, if the protocol requires obtaining dry ice for sending a sample to a laboratory, you should be able to inform the site visitors how you will secure it. In instances where we needed small amounts of dry ice, we occasionally would get it from the Good Humor Ice Cream vendor, as his route took him past our office twice a day.

This is a good time to again approach the issue of "outcome" and "process." Having a good outcome is essential to bring in repeat business. Your site must meet its allocated number of patients, and the work must be good. That is, the data needs to be clean, well supported and unquestionably accurate. This outcome must be consistent. Your site is only as good as the last study done there. This is why a site is better off not taking trials that place in question the site's ability to perform. It is far better not to take a study than to take it and to produce poorly. People will remember you as having a high level of integrity if you are honest about not being able to do a trial. They will come back. However, if you take a trial and fail, all that they will remember is your failure. It is unlikely they will return.

The other part of the equation is "process." This is best explained through an example. I had an experience with a limousine service where I was billed at more than three times the usual rate for a trip. Instead of the usual charge of $64, the charge was $212. I complained to the local billing clerk who was not receptive. I later complained to the local company manager who also refused to listen. Finally, days later, I complained to the regional manager who was very accommodating and receptive. He immediately credited me with the $212 and applied the appropriate charge of $64. The outcome here, ultimately, was good. The process, though, will keep me from ever using this limousine service again.

The same is true for your site. To be successful, to attract repeat business, you must make your process good. You must remember who the customer is in this relationship. It is difficult to keep this in mind because as an investigator, you are generally treated with so much respect that it is easy to lose perspective. You must remember that there are many investigators who would like to participate in the trial for which you have been selected. They also would like to receive the grant. So, you need to accommodate the monitors, clinical scientists and others who need to have questions resolved, visits made and generally be responded to in a brisk and preferential fashion.

The sites that remain successful in this business always remember that they have two customers: the sponsors and the subjects.

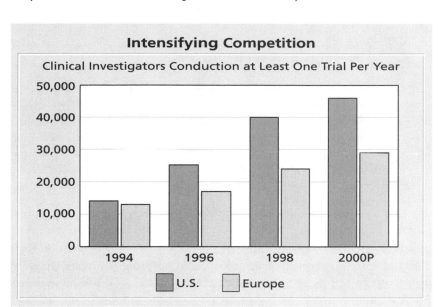

Source: CenterWatch, CMR

The growing competition for grants is forcing investigators and investigative sites to develop regular marketing efforts. All of the marketing strategies outlined above for the novice investigator can be employed by the experienced site as well. Most experienced sites will regularly write to pharmaceutical companies and CROs with whom they have not worked before and tap into industry publications for information about sponsors and CROs that will be starting new trials in the coming months. The common denominator is that all active, effective sites are continually looking for work. It is necessary to plan six months to a year in advance to keep a site continually busy. Here are some other ways that sites market themselves.

Wooing the Monitor
The monitor who periodically visits an investigative site during a trial is responsible for checking case report forms and generally reviewing the progress of the research. A monitor is a type of auditor, which can make the relationship between monitor and investigator an uneasy one. The experienced site, however, knows that the monitor frequently plays a key role in selecting investigators. A monitor who likes to come to a particular site will steer future grants to that site. Every time a monitor visits, a site has an opportunity to market itself.

The best way to court a monitor is with good work. The next best way is with simple courtesies. Make certain that the monitor has a comfortable work space. The study coordinator and investigator should make sure the monitor feels welcome at the site. Make sure the area is well equipped with fax and phone data ports. Coffee, soft drinks and access to a bathroom that is not used by patients are also good ideas.

It Helps if You Live in Vail

A site that is located in a desirable geographic location is going to have a leg up on the competition when it comes to securing grants. Often, the CRA who is going to do the monitoring will help select the sites. The monitor may visit each site as many as eight times over the course of a typical study. An investigator practicing in the mountains of Colorado is going to look very attractive as a site if the monitor is an avid skier. A site that is close to a major airport will also have an advantage. CRAs spend so much of their time traveling that anything that lessens their travel time to and from sites is considered a big plus.

Tracking Drugs in Development

There are currently more than 500 compounds in phase II studies. On average, about half of all compounds that enter phase II go on to be tested in phase III studies. The phase II pipeline usually produces more than 200 new compounds entering phase III research each year. By tracking drugs moving through the pipeline, a site can approach sponsors at the time they are seeking investigators for their large phase III trials.

Once a compound has been in a phase II study for a number of months, the pharmaceutical company will begin getting feedback on its safety and efficacy. If the initial results are promising, it will begin planning for phase III studies, even before the phase II work is completed. As part of this planning stage, it will begin gathering a pool of candidate investigators for the phase III research.

This is an ideal time for a site to write to the sponsor. In the next few months, the sponsor will be awarding grants to 25 to 50 investigators (or more). The sponsor is now actively looking for investigators. A site that identifies the appropriate contact person for the compound can send a letter specifically describing its relevant expertise and patient population. It is important, however, to write to the contact person, rather than call. A project leader at a pharmaceutical company can feel deluged by calls from investigative sites. As a result, a "cold call" can even work against a site.

A site that approaches sponsors in this timely manner, inquiring about participating in a study for a specific compound, will stand out as one that has done its homework. The site has taken the time and effort to make an informed pitch to the sponsor. There are several ways a site can become informed about drugs moving through the pipeline and contact sponsors prior to the initiation of phase III studies.

CenterWatch tracks drugs moving through phase I, phase II and phase III trials, and then, in each issue, publishes a list of sponsors and CROs who want to receive inquiries from investigators interested in participating in the next stage of research. Typically, each issue contains leads for 20 to 30 compounds.

A site can also develop its own tracking system by drawing on information from a variety of industry publications. Clinical Investigator News and Clinical Trials Monitor, which are published monthly by CTB International, both carry information about drugs in development. The Pink Sheet, which is published by F-D-C, provides a weekly update on the pharmaceutical industry.

Attending Industry Meetings and Conferences

Another common way that sites market themselves today is by attending industry-wide, annual meetings and conferences that focus on "site" issues. These annual meetings and conferences can provide excellent networking opportunities.

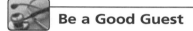 **Be a Good Guest**

Everyone recognizes that investigators' meetings are supposed to provide a mini-vacation opportunity. Please do not abuse the sponsor's hospitality. It will come back to haunt you in your quest for future work. Once, for example, I sent to a start-up meeting an investigator from one of our sites who, at the end of the meeting, decided to empty the mini-bar in his hotel room into his suitcase. I soon received a very irate call from the CRA monitoring his site. The investigator was asked to reimburse the sponsor $523 for the mini-bar charges. As you would expect, he never worked for that sponsor again.

The two best-known annual conferences are sponsored by the Drug Information Association (DIA) and the Association of Clinical Research Professionals (ACRP). The fee for joining these organizations is minimal, and you will receive regular mailings and the journals that they publish. Their annual meetings attract representatives from pharmaceutical companies, CROs and investigative sites, which make them a good forum for making new contacts.

There are now a number of for-profit companies that are organizing conferences related to the clinical research industry. There are at least four to five conferences each year that focus specifically on issues related to investigative sites. The conferences typically attract 50 to 100 people and last two to three days. Usually, it is a site's coordinator or business manager who attends the conference. The attendees typically are from dedicated research sites, SMOs and academic medical centers.

Attending Your Own Specialty Meetings

Frequently pharmaceutical companies attend meetings such as that of the American Heart Association with the specific agenda of identifying investigators for some new or on going trials. Speak to the individuals at the booths. Many times, they will be the specific individuals or will be able to point you to people who can get you involved. Again, in general, these individuals will differ from the marketing folks and will be at the conference for certain reasons. Try and find them.

Advertising at Industry Conferences
Many larger sites rent display booths at the annual meetings held by the Drug Information Association and ACRP. There is a significant cost to this type of marketing, and it is a strategy that is useful only for full-time dedicated research sites.

Advertising on the Internet
Another way to advertise your services is on the Internet. As mentioned earlier in this chapter, CenterWatch operates a web site (centerwatch.com) that has become a clearinghouse for information about clinical research. Pharmaceutical companies, CROs and investigative sites use it to recruit patients for their trials. In addition, the CenterWatch web site includes a directory of centers that conduct clinical research that sponsors and CROs can use to identify investigators by therapeutic specialty and geographic region. Each listing of an investigative site includes information about its facilities, experience, staff expertise and patient demographics. Two other web sites, Research Investigator's Source (clinicalinvestigators.com) and Clinmark (clinmark.com), also provide online directories of investigative sites.

Also, it is a good idea to build your own web site. Now, more than ever, the industry is communicating on the web. Include your Internet address on all information about your site and on your business card. This will facilitate communication from both sponsors and CROs.

The Initial Site Visit

Prior to awarding an investigator a grant, it is common practice for the pharmaceutical company, or the CRO representing it, to visit the investigative site. This initial site visit is an essential aspect of the good clinical practices mandated by the FDA. The purpose is to assure the sponsor that the site, in fact, exists, and that it has the necessary equipment and office space to conduct clinical research. This visit also provides an investigative site with an opportunity to impress a sponsor with its commitment to research.

Often, one of the people visiting the site is the clinical research associate (CRA) who will do the monitoring during the study. Frequently a clinical scientist or the medical monitor will also be present. Sometimes there is someone from quality assurance as well. You will not be awarded a grant unless these individuals have a positive feeling about your site and your ability to conduct the study. Your study coordinator must be present at the initial site visit.

Typically, the site visit will begin with a tour of the office. The CRA will have a checklist. Does the site have a locked storage space for the drug? (This is a federal requirement, and if you do not have it you will not get the grant.) Does the site have a file cabinet for storing study documents? Is there a waiting area for patients? If a study requires special equipment, does the site have it? For example, if a cardiogram is required as part of the protocol, the monitor will want to see the machine.

During this initial site visit, the CRA (or pharmaceutical representative) will want the site to identify a monitor work area. As you would expect, this is an important item on the checklist for a CRA. The monitor's work area should include adequate space, a desk, a phone and some privacy. A fax machine is a plus as is a data port. Close proximity to a refrigerator and a bathroom is also helpful. The CRA needs to be assured that during a monitoring visit, this space will be off-limits to others in the office.

Among CRAs, complaints about poor work areas at sites are a source of black humor. CRAs regularly tell of having to work in a waiting room, balancing their papers on their laps, while regular patients look on. An investigative site needs to think of the monitor as a client who will be a regular guest. An investigative site that has set up a nice work space for a monitor has gone a long way toward securing not only the immediate grant, but future grants as well.

At many pre-study visits, the site will be asked to show charts of patients who fit the protocol's inclusion-exclusion criteria. These charts should be pulled prior to the monitor's arrival. However, a site should not simply pull charts for patients who fit the general therapeutic category. A site should closely screen the charts and include only those that appear to fit the inclusion-exclusion criteria perfectly. If the CRA reviews your pulled charts and determines that many of the patients would not be good candidates, the CRA is likely to conclude that you haven't done your homework and that you won't pay proper attention to the study.

As you will have already reviewed the protocol, the initial site visit presents an opportunity for you to raise any questions you may have. Asking questions shows the monitor or visiting representative that you have thought about the challenges that will be presented by the trial. Also, anything you can do to show that you are familiar with the protocol's details will impress the monitor. For example, if the protocol requires a sample to be shipped in dry ice, a site should know how it will get the ice.

You will need to allocate time for the initial study visit. On average, it requires about one hour to one and a half hours of the investigator's time and perhaps two hours of the coordinator's time. Set this time aside so that neither you nor the study coordinator will be interrupted by patient visits or calls. This time commitment should be considered part of the cost of doing the study for which you will be ultimately reimbursed.

Both the investigator and study coordinator should radiate confidence about their site's ability to successfully conduct the study. The monitor wants to select sites that are confident they can perform. Your visitors will want to be assured that the site will be able to enroll and retain patients for the proposed study. If you express doubts about your ability to accomplish the goals, then they will choose a site other than yours.

6

C H A P T E R

Setting Up The Office

- Financing
- The Cash Flow Crunch
- Company Structure
- Facility
- Equipment
- Recruitment Center
- Office Costs

The most labor intensive approach to getting involved in clinical research is for you to set up shop as an independent investigative site. This, however, also ultimately confers the greatest degree of autonomy and profitability. No matter what route you choose, you will have to make some changes in the way you normally operate your practice and your office. Research will require changes in your office to accommodate research patients, monitors, additional equipment and secured storage for both drugs and files. If you go it alone, you will also have to build infrastructure to support what is essentially a separate business.

Once you and your group have decided that you want to become involved in clinical research, you will need to take a business-like approach to the entire process. This includes setting up a facility that enhances the conduct of trials, hiring or training the appropriate personnel, marketing your facility and producing quality, timely work.

It is particularly important to do things properly from the start. Set up systems that will demonstrate an effective and first-rate approach. Do not be short-sighted. Make sure that the physical, accounting, personnel and general support systems look like they are top-notch and also expandable. Look to the future. Project potential growth, and don't lock yourself into a situation that will not accommodate it.

Financing

As I mentioned above, if you are pursuing clinical research, it is best considered in the context of a business venture. Like all new businesses, this one will require some time to get out of the red. You must be prepared to carry an enterprise that might be negative in cash flow for up to 18 months, depending on how vigorously you approach this initiative. Actually, those people who are most successful are, in many ways, more likely to exhibit negative cash flow at the beginning than those physicians who do research in a more casual way. Ultimately, a little patience and foresight up front will result in large rewards down the road.

Do not under-capitalize your initiative. Lack of funds up front will simply create so much pressure that a new venture into clinical research will not get an adequate amount of time to prove itself. It will take between one and two years to begin to be in the black. This is because of the lengthy delays in payment, and the fact that during the first year, you will be constantly contributing new resources. However, there will be some income immediately upon acquiring your first trial.

All situations are different, but in an attempt to give some perspective, I will give some general guidelines about resource requirements. The novice investigator will have to invest in this process. How vigorously you intend to develop this component of a practice determines the amount of financing required. In general, the most common mistake physicians make in doing clinical research is that they under-capitalize themselves. Most physicians, for example, would never consider securing a line of credit specifically for this purpose. So, what they do is try to finance research out of their normal cash flow. Consequently, all components of the practice, including their own salaries, suffer from too little money. In the short run, this applies so much pressure to the practice that the initiative is never allowed to mature. It will probably take 18 months to begin to get a good flow of cash from this pipeline. But once it starts, you will never want to turn off the tap.

A credit line of $250,000 should, in almost all cases, give your venture enough funding to keep it from becoming burdensome to the other components of your organization and practice. A credit line is a good way to go because there is no sense paying interest on unnecessary capital. And, if things go slightly better than average, you may only need a small percentage of this money.

The Cash Flow Crunch

In the past, sponsors would commonly pay 25% or, occasionally, even more of the total budget up front. This payment was designed to cover the investigator's costs associated with preparing to start a study and getting to the point where the first patient could be enrolled. Today, these payments are much smaller. Sponsors may pay as little as 5% of the total budget or, even, not pay anything until the first patient is enrolled. Despite these declining up-front payments, the site still has to support an infrastructure that enables it to do trials. This infrastructure contains many fixed costs that do not increase whether the site does one trial or 15 trials. Of course, there are some increases in non-fixed costs, but the more trials you do, the more profitable they become.

The contract will then usually call for interim payments to be made during the course of the trial, based on the achievement of milestones, such as the number of patients randomized into the trial. Typically, the interim payments are not made until a monitor has visited the site and has confirmed that the milestone has been achieved. Even after the monitor's visit, it can take several months for the sponsor to process the payment. The monitor has to send a payment request to the clinical scientist who must OK it and send it on to the accounts payable department. In some companies, there are additional steps, and you can see that if, for example, an individual is tardy or on vacation, it is easy to simply extend the approval component of this process. Then, once the payment request reaches the accounts payable department, it could take a month or more to work its way through the normal procedure.

The final payment may be for as much as 35% of the total grant. It will be requested only after the study is cleaned up and "put to bed." This means that the sponsor has reviewed all the data, all queries addressed to the site have been answered, all unused drugs returned, and a close-out visit completed. Just scheduling all this can take months. As a result, sites can wait six or more months after completing a trial until they receive final payment.

It is also true that the more organizations the payment flows through, the longer it takes to get paid. If a CRO is involved, the check might be delayed depending on the contract signed between the organizations. Sometimes the CRO is totally in control of issuing these investigator grants so it doesn't necessarily take longer. It is worth mentioning at this time that an investigator does not make less if he or she works through a CRO. Generally, investigator grants are budgeted separately and are not free to contribute to a CRO's profit. This is, again, a general statement and not inviolate. But, if payment flows through an SMO, a network or a practice management organization, it is likely that there will be accumulative delays. In these cases, an investigator will certainly make less.

The slowness of payment is a well-known problem in the clinical research industry. Sites complain about it constantly. Sponsors and CROs constantly talk about developing new procedures to address the complaints, but the truth is, it is not a high priority for them. There are plenty of investigators who are willing to wait, and a smart investigator simply considers this part of the cost of doing business. This is an issue all investigators deal with, so expect to do so if you pursue clinical research.

The average payment for a clinical trial is about $50,000. Net profit on each trial climbs to 50% after the baseline costs are covered. If a site does more than three or four trials a year, then clinical research becomes increasingly profitable. Many sites that do clinical research as an adjunct to their practice do 20 or more trials each year. At this level, the net can easily approach $400,000 or $500,000. I defy you to tell me of another honest way to increase your practice's revenue by this extent, particularly in today's milieu.

Company Structure

There are many ways to incorporate research into your practice. The simplest is to consider clinical trials as another cash stream and to simply place all revenues into the general coffers. Likewise, all expenses can simply be paid out of the same general accounts. This eliminates the cost of setting up a new company and the increased accounting fees and baseline costs that any separate organization requires. However, in general, this is not my recommendation. It is particularly important to separate out the research component from the practice component if there are multiple partners involved in the practice. It is likely that some will be more enthusiastic about research than others. It seems logical, therefore, that at some time in the future, there may be differences in earnings based on productivity in clinical research.

It is usually best to structure a separate research corporation and to have that company pay the clinical practice for services provided. This is the format that ultimately will offer the greatest degree of flexibility to the participants. For example, it is an excellent idea to make a highly productive coordinator a partner in the research company. This will go a long way to assure that this valuable employee does not get picked off by a sponsoring company (a rather frequent happenstance) because he or she is part-owner of the company. However, it is unlikely that you would ever consider giving this individual part of your practice. The separation of the two corporate structures will allow this.

Also, you may want to distribute rewards based solely on participation in clinical research and not in other practice components. It may be easier to do so through a separate corporation. In fact, some of your partners may have no desire at all to be involved in research. A separate company gives you a mechanism for proceeding without disrupting a practice that might be functioning quite well.

Finally, there is currently a good market in productive trial sites. You might want to sell your trial site eventually without selling your practice. A little foresight will prevent all sorts of problems and will actually enhance your ability to sell the research component.

Delegate, Delegate

Participating in clinical research will not be worthwhile if the trials seriously interfere with the normal function of an investigator's office. The trick is to delegate all routine tasks to the study coordinator and other office staff. The investigator should only do those tasks that he or she is clearly, and unavoidably, expected to do. The vast majority of the work should be carried out by others. In my office, for example, the rule was that any physician who touched the case report form would have his or her thumbs broken.

The Facility

Before a pharmaceutical company will award a novice investigator a research grant, it will send a representative to visit the site. This is a federally mandated requirement.

A new investigator needs to take this initial site visit and turn it from a routine encounter into a marketing opportunity. Here is a chance to show the sponsor that you have a functioning, up-to-date facility that is structured to facilitate the accomplishment of their trials.

Packaging counts a lot here. A clean, modern facility with all the right components in place will go a long way to reassuring a sponsor or CRO that they want to do business with you. Most important, it will show them that you know what you are doing. One of a sponsor's worst nightmares is placing a trial in a site that has no understanding of how to get it done. Consequently, this first impression is critical, and the novice site needs to utilize it to score points.

Here is what a sponsor or CRO will look for:

A Dedicated Study Area

A pharmaceutical company wants to know that you consider clinical research as important, not just a casual adjunct to your practice, and you have made the investment to do it well. A specific, dedicated area for seeing study patients and conducting visits is absolutely necessary. This area is commonly the study coordinator's office.

A dedicated study office should be spacious enough to allow for the routine examination equipment including a table, cabinets, sink, and some office equipment. It may not be possible to include all this in one room, so it is quite OK to separate the examination room from the coordinator's business area. The facility needs to have a bright, cheerful and functional appearance.

The business component of this facility needs to have at least one phone line, preferably a fax machine, a data port, several comfortable chairs, a large desk, and locked storage cabinets (they should be locked, and the keys should not be dangling from the lock). A copy machine should be in the office or in close proximity. Additional shelving and/or large utility cabinets for storage of active case report forms should be present.

A dedicated study area should also have room for a computer station. There should be data ports for transmission of data. It is becoming more of a common requirement that investigators submit their data electronically to the CRO or sponsor. The computer itself and the modem line used for this remote data entry will always be paid for and installed by the sponsor. An investigative site that is doing multiple studies at the same time will have a separate computer for each trial. Every CRO and sponsor, by the way, jealously guards their own remote data entry system when they have one. Consequently, your coordinator might find himself or herself using multiple software packages at the same time.

The location of your study facility should not be too far off the physician investigator's routine beaten path. He or she will have to see the study patients to do physicals and the other investigative parts of the visits. Generally, these interactions are brief, so if it takes the investigator longer to walk to the study area than to do the examination, it is not a productive use of his or her time. Also, coordinators will have questions and require support.

Another important reason for situating the study area close to the patient care area is that there are certain studies that require the practice to fuel them. An example would be a study involving a new antibiotic for the treatment of strep throat. In this instance, either the coordinator or the patient would have to relocate because entrance into the study could not be pre-planned. It was my practice to have the coordinator take all materials necessary to enter the patient to the examination room and to do the first visit right there. I had already done a physical as part of my routine visit, so the process flowed very smoothly. However, if the coordinator had to transverse a large distance to make it to the patient in the examination room it is likely that this would have an impact on overall patient flow throughout the entire office. This is even more likely because the coordinator always had to retrieve some items from her office that she had forgotten initially.

Another issue worth mentioning is that you and your coordinator should leave exposed only those things that you want the sponsor or CRO to see. If you leave confidential material dealing with other trials out, then the visiting inspectors will assume that you will do the same with their confidential material. Also, you may not want the CRO or sponsor to know what other studies you are doing currently or how many. In this case, do not leave lists or charts in places where visitors will find them.

A Waiting Room for Study Volunteers

A physician in practice is providing a service to his or her patients. Although it is important to have an attractive, pleasant waiting room, the patients understand that what is of utmost importance is the care and time they receive from the physician. But as a clinical researcher, your relationship to your patient is quite different. In a sense, the patient is providing you with a service. The patient is volunteering for a trial, and by doing so, is enabling you to generate a fee from the pharmaceutical company. One way to show your appreciation to study volunteers – provided you have the space – is to set up a "study volunteers only" waiting room.

 Where Have All the Patients Gone?

One trial required that patients be fed measured, high-fat diets for three days, have serum lipid levels every 90 minutes and be monitored continually, to ensure compliance, for the entire 72-hour period. The trial began in July, and we divided the volunteers into two groups of 12 each. We had the facility at the office to sleep that many and also a kitchen to prepare the food. The study was conducted over the weekend so as to not interfere with work schedules. One Sunday morning of that particularly hot July, I drove to the site to make sure all was going well. When I got there, I couldn't find any of my coordinators or the patients. I quickly drove to the in-charge coordinator's home, and there I found all the patients and coordinators enjoying themselves in her pool. The scene that I will never forget is 12 patients swimming in her pool, each of them keeping the arm with the intercath extended above their heads.

This might seem like one of those things you would like to have but that should be put off until the clinical trial concept begins to prove itself. Actually, it is very important for several reasons. The first is that, again, packaging counts, and if you set your site up so that it looks like a very functional, well equipped site, then it will further your attempts to solicit work.

The second issue is that many studies require that the patient spend some large blocks of time in the office. Sometimes it is required that they have their vital signs checked hourly, other times diary information is collected every hour, and sometimes it is other things. So, having an appropriate place for you to house the subjects will allow you to participate in a wide variety of trials.

Finally, a dedicated waiting room sends the correct message to your trial patients. It makes them feel as if they are members of a highly valued group. This is one way of encouraging current trial patients to participate in future studies and also to subliminally suggest participation to others in your practice. On a more pragmatic front, having a separate waiting room will keep study patients from congesting your practice waiting room.

The dedicated waiting area should be furnished with comfortable chairs or recliners so that a patient might even doze undisturbed for a few hours.

It is a good idea to keep it stocked with a variety of reading material including daily papers, magazines and novels. It is a good idea to have a VCR and a TV along with a selection of tapes for people to watch. Also, a coffee maker, a small refrigerator stocked with some juice and soft drinks, and a box of doughnuts are nice.

This may seem as if you are overdoing things a little but the patient is the ultimate coinage in the world of clinical research. These are the individuals who make you successful and if you treat them well, it is amazing the distance they will go to ensure their successful participation.

Locked Drug Storage

Federal regulations require a clinical investigator to have a secure, lockable storage area for trial drugs. Be assured that this is one of the things that will be looked at when your site is visited. Some professional sites have built-in storage rooms for study drugs and have outfitted them with alarm systems and fire retarding systems to ensure the safety of the drugs. As long as you have a padlocked closet or storage cabinet, this should suffice. It is best to keep the drugs locked up in close proximity to your coordinators, since they will be the ones doing the dispensing and drug inventories. In fact, it was my habit to lock the drug in the office of the coordinator doing the trial.

Production of sample material for clinical trials is a very costly process so samples are distributed frugally. Today, many sponsors have instituted "just in time" supply systems utilizing telephone access coding and a centralized distribution system. One of the things this does for the site is to reduce the amount of space required for drug storage. However, more is always better than less here, and this should not be an issue for anyone. Just set this up in advance so you can actually show it to those who visit to qualify your site. Otherwise you are not going to be judged an appropriate site.

Record Storage Area

Clinical trials generate a large amount of paper. During a trial, you will want to keep your case report forms in file cabinets or shelves located in the coordinator's study office. But, once a trial is complete, you will want to clear all this material out to allow space for new trials. A remote storage facility, somewhere that occupies less premier space at your site or even in a remote location, is the ticket. The need to store this material varies according to the stage of the trial and the company you work for. Some companies state that you must hold everything until you receive a letter from them allowing you to discard materials. Others state that you must hold everything for two years after approval. Other companies tell you to hold everything indefinitely. One of my rules of clinical trials is, "don't ever throw anything away." I hold all files indefinitely.

When a study is complete, the normal process is for the coordinator and monitor to collect all case report forms, all dispensing and monitoring logs, and all other documentation including IRB correspondence and to seal it jointly in banker boxes. This material then needs to be stored in a place where it can be retrieved with a few days' notice in case of an FDA audit. And, it is not uncommon for these audits to occur several years after the trial has been completed.

Patient Database
If your practice has a functional database that enables you to sort your patient population according to disease states, current medications and demographics, then you have a device that will help you attract trials. If, during this initial site visit you can demonstrate this potential, you will find that people who visit will frequently call when they are assessing the feasibility of future trials. This feasibility assessment designates the earliest possible involvement for an investigator, and this is exactly where in the process you want to be considered.

A Monitor Work Area
During a trial, you will be monitored routinely by the sponsor or CRO. The monitor who visits you will come to visit according to his or her schedule, your rate of enrollment and the importance and complexity of the protocol. The monitor will check the case report forms, the drug inventory and the source documents. Source documentation, by the way, is a major consideration in doing good clinical research. Essentially, what is documented in the case report form needs to be verified and supported by other clinical records. For example, there must be progress notes that support patient visits. We will talk more about this in the regulatory section, but suffice it to say that part of what a monitor does is to check the case report forms against the source documentation to ensure there are no discrepancies.

You can see that the monitors spend a lot of time at the sites doing very tedious work. It makes good sense, then, to provide a facility where they are comfortable and can function effectively. And, if I were a monitor, one reason why I might choose one site over another was that I could better accomplish my job at one of them.

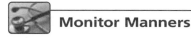 **Monitor Manners**

On many occasions, I have discussed working conditions with friends who work as monitors (CRAs). It never ceases to amaze me how rudely they are treated by some sites. One friend told me that the only space allocated to her when monitoring a particular site was the restroom. Other CRAs have told me that they have had to work in waiting rooms, and do all their work without the benefit of a desk or any privacy whatsoever. A site that does not provide adequate work space for monitors is antagonizing the very people who will help determine whether it will be awarded future grants.

Many sites fail to appreciate the importance of wooing the monitors. Monitors often complain of coming to sites where they are forced to sit or even stand in cramped space, or at a makeshift table, to get their work done. Sites fail to provide them with access to a phone, data port, fax and copier. They are treated as annoyances as opposed to important colleagues.

The monitor is the sponsor's (or CRO's) eyes and ears. The monitor is the person who gains a hands-on impression of the reliability and quality of your site and of whether you should be selected to conduct future trials. Monitors do, more or less frequently depending upon the company, play an important role in site selection. As such, from a business perspective, it is essential that the monitor be treated with consideration. Think of every monitor visit as an opportunity to sell your site to that company.

Some companies hire free-lance monitors. These individuals work for multiple companies, and a good relationship with one of them can translate into work for many different companies. If the monitor wants to work at your site, if you make his or her life easier, then it is likely your site will be advanced at every company he or she works for.

As you set up your office, make sure that you provide the monitor with a pleasant work space. A well-lit desk, a comfortable chair, phone and fax access as well as a place to hook his or her computer into the sponsor's network are important. Make sure that the monitor has access to coffee and soft drinks and is provided with the means either to buy lunch or to join your staff at lunch. It was always my policy to treat the monitor and coordinator to lunch in-house or at an area restaurant.

Monitors are like everyone else: they want to work in a friendly atmosphere. Create that warm and friendly environment and you will have a good chance that the monitor will return to your office every chance he or she gets.

Conference Room

This is a terrific asset if you have the space for one. This room will get frequent use at study initiation visits, study close-outs and during company-sponsored audits. It is a great venue in which the investigator can introduce himself or herself and the staff to potential clients.

Equipment

A clinical trial site needs equipment to carry out the medical procedures required by the protocols in which the site agrees to participate. If, for example, a pulmonary function study is required in an asthma trial, then the machine needs to be available for inspection during the initial site visit. There is some general equipment that would be worth purchasing up front. This includes a minus 70 degrees freezer, a good mercury sphygmomanometer, a good scale and other general medical equipment.

Frequently, the company supplies you with specific medical equipment, and, usually, the equipment is donated to the site at the termination of the trial. I received a variety of medical and office equipment that was put to good use in my medical practice. These included 24-hour blood pressure monitoring equipment, a minus 70 degrees freezer, a variety of fax machines and other office equipment. The sponsoring companies tend to be very generous in this manner because it is almost as costly and quite a bit more trouble to reclaim the equipment. This works out to be a very nice additional incentive for the site.

The Sweet Smell of Success

The trial involved the testing of a new drug that caused weight loss by inhibiting intestinal lipase. One of the ways that we were measuring the effectiveness of the product was through 72-hour fecal fat measurements. The sponsoring company donated huge freezers to the sites to accommodate the massive amount of material collected. The only lab certified to make the analysis was in Sweden, and the material had to be collected and then shipped in bulk for analysis. This all worked quite well until my site lost electric power because of a severe winter storm. I vowed to get a back-up generator for the next trial, because it took a long time until any of us could comfortably use the section of the office where the freezer resided.

Recruitment Center

A new investigative site will probably draw most of the patients directly from the investigator's practice to fill the trials with which the site becomes involved. It is easy to supplement the flow of patients with ads placed in local papers, posters at community centers and other basic forms of advertisement. Some of the more sophisticated sites have installed fully computerized telephone soliciting systems manned 18 hours a day in order to "cold call" for study participation and to construct a large patient database. This type of system generally requires at least a room 10 feet by 10 feet. The equipment is expensive and the commitment large, so I would suggest not investing in this type of set-up until you are certain of your long-term interest in clinical research.

Office Costs

Here is a sample list of costs associated with setting up an office for clinical research. These figures do not include the cost of office space for a waiting room, or an examination room for seeing clinical research patients.

Exam Room

Exam table	$750
Desk	500
Locked Cabinet	500
Fax	350
Two chairs	300
Phone and phone line	250
	$2,650

Waiting Room

Furniture	$2,500
TV/VCR	750
Coffee maker	50
	$3,300

Total	**$5,950**

7

The Study Coordinator

- Education
- Finding the Coordinator
- Training
- Personality
- Retaining a Study Coordinator
- Hiring a Second Study Coordinator
- Other Staff

W hen sponsors and CROs select a site for participation in a trial, they put a premium on the investigator's experience and expertise. But, there is also an oft-repeated truism in the clinical trial industry that "the most important individual at the investigative site is not the investigator. It is the study coordinator."

This is true in other regions of the world as well. The coordinator has crossed the Atlantic. As the Europeans embrace clinical trials in a more commercial fashion, the adoption of the medical coordinator job is probably the major innovation that is accelerating the development of European trial sites.

Probably the most critical decision you will make as a clinical investigator deals with the selection of appropriate study coordinators. The study coordinator runs the trial. A coordinator also can help manage all other aspects of the trial business. For example, it is not unusual for coordinators to market a site, secure the grants, be involved with the accounting, structure budgets, and pay patient stipends. A coordinator frequently does all these things in addition to his or her primary responsibility of actually running the trial. This all depends, of course, on how involved you as an investigator wish to be and how sophisticated a system you wish to install.

The primary responsibility of the coordinator must remain the hands-on control of the trial. This begins prior to the actual start of the trial. In fact, there is a lot of up-front work involved. First is the careful and complete understanding of every component of the trial including the documentation required. Much of this is discussed at the start-up meetings, so it is absolutely necessary that a coordinator attend these (someone who is afraid to fly could not be considered for this job). Other things must be dealt with prior to the start of the trial, including arranging for clinical laboratory pickups, monitoring visits, and other mechanical issues. This could be as simple as finding a source for dry ice.

Then, of course, there is dealing with the regulatory issues. The coordinator generally puts together the IRB submission. Included in the package sent to the IRB is the 1572, all CVs, the consent form, the protocol, the drug manual and any advertisements that are to be used to attract patients. As the study progresses, the coordinator keeps the IRB updated.

The coordinator also is the interface between your site and the pharmaceutical company or CRO. It is the coordinator who deals, almost on a daily basis, with the CRA. It is the coordinator who responds to all queries and resolves them. It is the coordinator who is present for every monitoring visit and reviews all the data with the monitor because the coordinator is the individual who fills out the case report forms. This is one of the essential elements of the job. The coordinator must be able to consistently follow instructions and to correctly record into the case report forms. This does not seem like something that should cause a great deal of difficulty, but, the truth is, it is remarkable how few people can consistently follow instructions.

Another major component of the coordinator job is dealing with the patients. Most times the coordinator is intimately involved in the recruitment process as well as in every patient visit as required by the protocol. This individual must be able to keep the subjects on the right path and to make sure that the patient remains compliant. At the same time, the coordinator must be constantly vigilant for any adverse effects because the investigator will not see the patient on every visit.

Drug dispensing and inventory is another component of the job. It is normally the coordinator who assumes this critical task in the research trial. This frequently includes calculating dosage and dosing schedules. Clearly, at least basic math skills are a must.

If you select the right person to be your coordinator and nurture that relationship, your participation in clinical research will be an emotional pleasure and financially rewarding. If you don't, you will quickly find that clinical research is a chore, too demanding and a financially unattractive enterprise.

Here are some of things you need to consider when selecting a coordinator:

Education

The study coordinator position has no specific educational requirements. There is nothing that says a coordinator has to have a medical background at all. Some investigators enlist current employees, their wives or others to train in this position. They may prove to be ideally suited for the job. There are, of course, certain types of training that would be advantageous to the position.

Medical training is an asset. In fact, the higher the level of medical capability, the better. The more a coordinator is able to do on his or her own, without the investigator, the better the trial will flow. That is, if the coordinator needs to find an investigator each time a pulse or blood pressure measurement is needed, then there will obviously be long delays for the patient as well as much useless energy expended simply locating people and then waiting for the completion of simple tasks. The most frequent background for a coordinator is nursing. An RN, in many ways, has ideal training for this position. The medical training of this individual brings an additional level of safety to the entire study process. By this I mean that during most visits required in a clinical trial, very few will necessitate investigator-patient interactions. Consequently the entire visit is conducted by the coordinator. This means that if that coordinator has a high level of medical sophistication, then subtle adverse events or inter-current medical problems are more likely to be recognized. In fact, another ideal background for a coordinator is that of physician. There are many unlicensed foreign physicians living in the United States today who are looking for work. Many of these physicians have no expectations of ever practicing in the United States. Being a coordinator seems to be an ideal position for someone in such a circumstance.

Others with excellent medical backgrounds include physician assistants. The advantage here is that the PA can be listed as a sub-investigator on the 1572 form (This form, which is required for each clinical trial, will be discussed more in chapter nine. On it must be listed all individuals who are participating in the conduct of the trial). This allows the PA to conduct almost every visit without the investigator being required to interrupt his or her schedule at all.

This does not mean that coordinators without formal medical training cannot do an excellent job. Many do, and they learn the necessary techniques to function effectively in this role. Some sites actually prefer to train non-medical people because of the expense of hiring RNs.

Other background elements that could prove helpful include some computer training. Today, many trials require remote data entry by the site, so a familiarity with computers would be an advantage here. If a coordinator has the ability to set up computerized systems to track progress in trials and payments, it could be of great added value to the site. This also applies to abilities to structure web sites and to create initiatives on the web.

People bring very diverse backgrounds to this position, and this can enable them to contribute in unique ways. For example, I know of a coordinator who has a graphic arts background. She uses her skills to help her site develop innovative and eye-catching patient recruitment ads.

One approach for a site might be to collect a variety of special skills as the site builds a team of coordinators, so that each set of individual strengths contribute to the others.

Finding the Coordinator

It is quite common for an investigator to have a specific individual in mind for this position even prior to establishing the initiative. Most times there is someone working in the investigator's practice or that he or she knows at the hospital who has the capabilities to do this job and is looking for a change in circumstances. This may even be the spouse of the future investigator. By far, this is the most common way of identifying an individual for this job, and it may be one of the better ones. It seems to me that you never know how a new employee is going to work out until you have spent six months working with him or her. This approach eliminates this question because it is likely that the individual in mind is someone who has worked with you for years. Do not discount the importance of good chemistry between the coordinator and investigator because it is surely one of the keys for building a good organization.

If this is not an option, then advertise for the appropriate individual. Specify the appropriate set of skills and suggest that experience as a clinical coordinator is a real plus. You might get lucky. There might be someone available or interested in making a change who brings a wealth of experience to the job. And, with this experience comes a series of connections into the industry that can jumpstart the site. By the same token, someone with a bad reputation will stifle growth, and it would be difficult for a novice investigator to recognize that this was happening until too late. So, check references carefully and check 10 of them, not just three. Make sure some are from CRAs at CROs and companies she or he has worked for. Finding an experienced coordinator can rocket a site on its way.

Training

There are multiple opportunities for coordinator training, both formal and informal. Sometimes the informal opportunities are the best. If you have a colleague or a friend who is involved in research, send your newly-hired coordinator to spend a month living at that site. There is nothing that will bring this individual up to speed quicker. In fact, there is nothing better than hands-on experience.

Many of the CROs have begun to run coordinator training courses. Both Parexel and Covance, who recently merged, run them in conjunction with some local colleges. These are excellent courses, and they are advertised in local papers prior to their start. Also, Barnett International runs frequent training courses. Barnett may be contacted at:

- **Barnett International**
  (800) 856-2556

The Association of Clinical Research Professionals (ACRP) is an organization that has a strong coordinator orientation, and they conduct both training and certifying examinations for coordinators. One of the prerequisites for the coordinator exam is that the coordinator be actively working in that occupation for at least two years before sitting for the exam. Actually it is an excellent idea for a site coordinator to be certified because that gives some reassurance to both sponsors and CROs that there is a certain basic level of knowledge and interest.

- **Association of Clinical Research Professionals (ACRP)**
  (202) 737-8100

Personality

A good coordinator is a jack-of-all-trades. The study coordinator must be able to handle a mix of medical, administrative, business, computer, patient and marketing chores. The following are some personality traits that seem to be common in good coordinators. It would be worth looking for these in an individual whom you are considering for the position.

First, a study coordinator must be a meticulous, detail-oriented individual. In today's parlance, this individual needs to be a "type A" personality. Your site will be judged on two primary indices. The first is productivity, and your coordinator will probably be very much involved in recruitment strategies and their execution. But the other index is cleanliness and accuracy of data, and it is entirely impossible to perform well here with out the concerted effort of the right coordinator. As previously mentioned, the collection of the data, the transfer of the data to the case report forms, and the resolution of queries are all a primary coordinator function. Queries are issued when there is a question or discrepancy involving submitted data. For example, if the birthdate on two separate forms, for the same patient, records that that individual is 42 years old on one and 24 years old on the other, then this would result in a data query. Not only does this slow the process of the study when the sponsor or CRO has to clean up inordinate numbers of these, they are expensive to correct. It is estimated that each time a query is issued, it costs almost $100 to get it resolved because it occupies the time of several employees and results in the generation of multiple forms. It also is expensive for the site because instead of a coordinator productively adding new patients to trials, she or he is bogged down in cleaning up old stuff that does not add to the bottom line. Sloppy work costs everybody, and the CROs frequently rate a site using a value derived from that site's rate of queries compared to other sites participating in the same trial. It is remarkable how widely these vary depending on the quality of the site. Meticulous attention to detail is at the heart of a coordinator's job, and the individual hired to do this job must approach life in this manner.

The Study Coordinator's Responsibilities Include...

- Marketing and networking with sponsors and CROS
- Protocol assessment
- Preparing and negotiating budgets
- Managing Sponsor and vendor payments
- Site preperation (e.g., training staff, obtaining IRD documents)
- Study coordination (e.g., recruiting, screening and scheduling patients, securing informed consent, study conduct)
- Case report form management
- Source documentation
- Test article inventory and accountability
- Adverse event reporting
- Study close-out

Source: ACRP

Another major component of a coordinator's job is working with the patients in the trial. The reason that many patients enter and remain in trials is because of the relationship they develop with the coordinator. The coordinator serves a function half-way between therapist, physician and mother to many of these individuals. It is typical for patients who have been discharged from a trial to continue to return for years simply to chat with the coordinator. The bond developed here is unbelievably strong and is incredibly helpful to the study process. I have personally seen patients go to remarkable lengths to help a coordinator get his or her job done. A coordinator who is good with patients will inspire them to complete the study and sign up for future ones. Also, the therapeutic value of these 30-minute, monthly sessions is of incalculable value to the patients.

The other major interaction a coordinator is involved with is between the coordinator and the CRAs. When a CRA visits, he or she will spend the majority of his or her time in company with the coordinator. If the relationship is good, the CRA will be interested in returning with future work. Friendships are built here and span the study relationship. These friendships are very valuable to the site. On the other hand, if there is constant tension and an uncomfortable atmosphere existing between the study coordinator and the CRA, then it is extremely unlikely that that CRA is likely to return to your site. A study coordinator who is warm and friendly and has good telephone skills is going to serve as an excellent salesperson for your site.

Another trait that would be advantageous in a study coordinator is creativity. The best coordinators look at protocols and find all sorts of ways to stay within their guidelines and still satisfy the needs of the patients and staff. They twist and turn the protocol without damaging it. They also devise methods to carry out their tasks that enable the process. Each protocol requires similar creative activities to make sure that it flows properly because each protocol has a unique set of problems and issues that have to be dealt with and overcome. A good site, investigator and coordinator will always find a way.

Finally, this individual must work well with the rest of your staff. There is nothing as disruptive as introducing a prima donna into a stable work environment. A team player, but more accurately, a team leader and builder is what you want to put into place.

Retaining a Study Coordinator

Once you have a good study coordinator, you have won half the staffing battle. The other half is keeping your coordinator. Because good coordinators are the types of individuals they are, they are frequently wooed by pharmaceutical companies and CROs to join their team with very good jobs as monitors. It is a common career path, and it is difficult for a small site to place offers that are competitive with those well-loaded, high-paying positions. In general, when "big pharma" calls, it is tough for a coordinator to say no. As you might expect, losing a good coordinator can prove devastating to a site. In essence, a site has suddenly lost the one person who runs its clinical research business. Unless a site is proactive, it can find itself scrambling to replace this loss.

Today, salaries for coordinators range from $55,000 to $85,000. Conventional wisdom states that to move someone normally requires a 15% increase in salary. Sponsoring companies can easily put that on the table, if they wish to make an offer. Also, they fully load their offers with generous health care, profit sharing, pension and vacation.

It is imperative to create a relationship with your coordinator that will help her or his retention as an employee of the site. One component of this offer is, of course, fiscal. First pay the right salary, and make sure there are incentives and bonuses. Share the wealth.

Second, consider sharing the research company. Create a partnership with your coordinator. This not only gives the coordinator tremendous upside potential if the site is sold in the future, but it also conveys the right message. Of course, to own a portion of this corporation, there will be stipulations that one must be employed by the corporation. It is likely that if you give up some stock, you will be rewarded with a different type of behavior than what is typical of an employee. Even though your coordinator, in an employee mode, is likely to give you 100% of his or her effort, it does not compare to the commitment that is typical of the owners of small business, exactly the type of behavior you should attempt to solicit. Consider putting 5% or 10% of the company on the table. If it makes you more comfortable, incorporate your research company in a state like Delaware where you can issue a class A voting stock to yourself and a class B, non-voting stock, to everyone else.

A third consideration is that people, in general, do not work for money alone. There are multiple intangibles that keep employees committed to their job. These include a sense of accomplishment and pride in their work, relationships at the office, a sense that they are appreciated, flexibility of a job and finally, that they have some measure of control over their own lives. All these things are contingent upon the tone set by the investigator. If these issues are considered frequently, and the atmosphere at the site is such that people are happy to go to work, then the chances of having your important employees cherry-picked is much less likely.

Hiring a Second Study Coordinator

Once you have secured your first few grants, you should consider hiring a second study coordinator. Then, the two coordinators working at your site can work out a coverage arrangement so that one is always available. This is particularly important for trials involving acute conditions.

A trial for an acute condition requires that volunteers be enrolled into the trial on the same day that they initially come to the office for treatment. An example of a study of this nature would be one comparing an investigational antibiotic to an approved antibiotic for treatment of strep throat infections. The patient must be enrolled into the trial at the time he or she presents at the office with the acute throat infection.

In this type of trial, it is less disruptive to your normal patient care paradigm if a trained coordinator is available to counsel the patient about enrolling into the trial. Here is how the interaction between physician and study coordinator would work. The physician would treat the patient in the normal fashion until there was confirmation of a positive, rapid strep test. At that moment, the physician would ask the patient if he or she would be interested in entering a trial comparing an investigational drug with a standard one. If the patient expressed interest, the physician would then explain the patient would have to review and sign a consent form that detailed all potential risks, that there would be no charge for the office visit and medication, that a small stipend would be paid to the patient (around $25 to $50), and that the patient would be required to return for a follow-up visit. If the patient is interested, and appears to fit the inclusion-exclusion criteria, the physician would then call in the study coordinator and go on to his or her next patient. The physician would have spent only five to 10 additional minutes in the exam room.

The coordinator would then take 30 minutes or so to carefully review with the patient the inclusion and exclusion criteria and the consent form. After the patient has reviewed the consent form, the physician returns and must then inquire whether the patient has any questions about either the consent form or the trial. The physician must confirm in writing, on the patient's chart, that he or she, as the investigator or sub-investigator, has indeed done this. Also it is necessary to document in the patient chart (source document) that the physician and the patient signed the consent form. The investigator can also check off the history and physical form because he or she has already obtained all this information even prior to asking the patient to enter the trial (as part of the routine examination). Once the patient agrees to participate in the trial, the study coordinator could obtain any required blood, urine and culture specimens and would dispense the drug and schedule the return visit.

If this is all done properly, the physician would have spent about 15 minutes with the patient, and the coordinator will have spent about one hour. At the follow-up visit, the physician would probably have to obtain a throat culture and just do an ears, nose and throat exam. The coordinator would have to spend about 30 minutes with the patient and, sometime that day, spend about another hour on the paperwork. The sponsor's payment to the site for this patient would be between $1,000 and $1,500 dollars.

So, because you can participate more effectively in a multitude of trials, but also because your organization does not become secure until you have done so, it is important to take on a second coordinator as soon as possible. That old adage about "not putting all your eggs in one basket" certainly applies here. In fact, many productive sites have between five and 15 full-time coordinators. It is also possible, with multiple coordinators, to assign a back-up for every ongoing trial, so that if someone leaves or is sick, the study will not suffer.

Other Staff

As you find yourself getting increasingly busy, and after you have hired at least several additional coordinators, there may be a variety of individuals whom it is appropriate to hire. For example, it may be possible to hire assistance for the coordinator to increase the number of trial each can maintain from eight to 12. Also, at some point, people specifically dedicated to patient recruitment and someone to market your site to the industry may eventually be worth hiring. You will know exactly when to do all these things because by the time these needs arises, you will have become highly sophisticated in this arena.

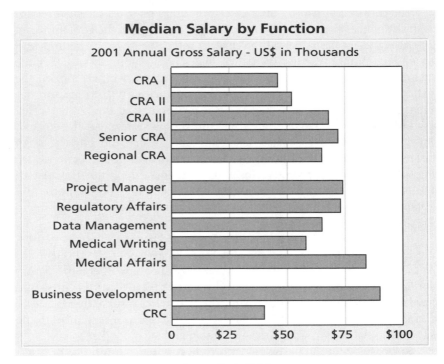

Source: CenterWatch

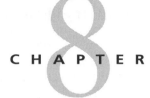

CHAPTER 8

The Study Initiation Process

Once a sponsor or CRO begins identifying sites for a trial, the study start-up process begins unfolding in a fairly rapid fashion. For a site, this study initiation process involves a number of steps. In order to run a profitable investigative site, it is essential that you devote attention to each of these steps. You especially need to critically review the protocol and proposed budget.

The Feasibility Process

Many CROs and a few sponsors do extensive feasibility surveys prior to the initiation of the study. These surveys are sent to investigators, identified through databases or the personal knowledge of those involved in the process. Normally, a brief confidentiality form proceeds the feasibility questionnaire. This form requests that the investigator give his or her opinion of the "real world" potential of actually accomplishing the trial. Do the inclusion and exclusion criteria prohibit enrollment? Do the patients called for in the protocol really exist? How many patients could the investigator supply and in what time frame?

You need to devote about a half hour of your time to answering these questions. There is seldom any reimbursement to you for your time and effort in completing this survey. However, it is certainly worth a half hour of your time because, sometimes, your effort is rewarded with a slot in the trial. As I have mentioned before, this does not always happen because at many sponsors and CROs, there is no connection between the people who collect feasibility information and those who actually place the trial. However, if you notice that your efforts are never rewarded with the trial at a particular company, you can simply not do feasibility work for that company.

The Initial Contact

There are two ways that a sponsor or CRO will initiate contact with investigative sites when looking to place a trial. One way is to fax a survey to potential sites. The survey will give a very brief description of the proposed trial and then inquire about the site's interest in doing the trial, its previous research experience and its patient demographics. This is a slightly different survey than the one for the feasibility process. The sponsor or CRO expects a site to return this survey within 24 to 48 hours. It is important, if the site is truly interested in doing the trial, that the responses are very positive. All the other sites who are receiving this initial survey are claiming to be able to enroll an enormous number of patients in a very short time frame. Nobody really believes them, and the common wisdom prevalent at CROs and sponsors suggests that you take whatever the response is and cut it in half. However, it is still clear that the sites that get chosen are those who promise the most. Consequently, if you return a survey that shows any hesitancy or reflects any uncertainty about your ability to accomplish the trial, your site will never be chosen. The only thing you must remember is that you might actually be held to what you say when you get the trial. You can see that it is necessary to walk a pretty fine line here. Be a bit conservative until your level of experience enables you to predict to a finer level. Remember, it still is the worst scenario to get a trial and then perform below expectations.

The second way to initiate contact is simply through a phone call in which the sponsor or CRO will inquire about the site's interest in the trial and ask for information about its experience and patient database. The same rules as above hold true here. If you want the trial, don't hedge your response with "maybe" and "probably." Go for it, and exude a convincing level of confidence. Otherwise, you will never get the trial.

After the initial contact is made, the site must sign a confidentiality agreement before it will be given an opportunity to review the study protocol. The pharmaceutical industry is very serious about this aspect of the research. Companies are frequently racing each other to the market with similar products, or with "me-too" products designed to compete with popular ones already on the market. In this environment, industrial espionage is a reality. An investigator contacted for a study will need to sign the agreement and abide by it.

Reviewing the Protocol

Once an investigator returns the confidentiality agreement, the company will send the study protocol by express mail. The document is the blueprint for the study. It details, step by step, what the investigator will have to do. It specifies inclusion-exclusion criteria. It provides information about the drug. You must review the protocol very carefully. The investigative site needs to determine whether this is a study it wants to do, whether it is a study it can do, and whether it is a study that is acceptable in relation to patient-care concerns. Reviewing the protocol carefully is also an essential first step toward negotiating an acceptable budget.

Accompanying the protocol will be a drug manual. This manual details all the known information accumulated in human and animal trials to date. It is very important that you read and digest this document carefully before making any decision about your participation in the trial. If you have any discomfort after reading this manual, consider seriously whether you want to participate in this trial. An investigator cannot effectively recruit for a study if he or she has a lot of questions about the benefit and safety of the product. You are better off saying no up front. It is always all right to say no.

In most cases, the drug will not appear to present any unusual risk to the patient. Often, the investigational drug will be similar to others of the same class that are already on the market. Or, the trial may be of a drug already on the market that the pharmaceutical company is testing for a new indication. Most physicians will be comfortable testing drugs of this type. As I've said before, any respectable pharmaceutical company will not be upset with an investigator that rejects a protocol because of safety concerns. That is feedback they should value and respect.

The next question an investigator needs to ask is whether the protocol can be done. Is it realistic? Most protocols are not constructed by practicing physicians, but by staff at the pharmaceutical company. The protocol needs to be "reality tested."

The reality test involves two components. First, are the inclusion-exclusion criteria realistic? Second, does the trial require too much of patients? Will patients be willing to volunteer for this protocol? The inclusion-exclusion criteria describe who is eligible to enter the study. There will be no exceptions to these criteria, unless an amendment is made to the protocol. A patient who is "close" to meeting the criteria cannot be enrolled. Are there patients who could meet the strict inclusion criteria?

For example, consider a protocol for an antidepressant that does not permit enrollment of anyone who has ever been treated with an antidepressant. That is an exclusion criterion that will make enrollment next to impossible. You should probably turn down this study. An investigator who tries to do this study will incur all the expenses associated with starting a study and will be unable to generate the per-patient fees stipulated in the contract. Furthermore, the sponsor may even complain that you are a site that is poor at patient enrollment.

In contrast, consider a protocol for an antidepressant that has less stringent exclusion criteria. This protocol does not permit enrollment of patients that have been on other antidepressants in the previous six months. Although that might exclude many patients, it is not an exclusion criterion that makes the study impossible to do. This protocol passes the reality test.

An investigator can evaluate inclusion-exclusion criteria by pulling patient charts. Do you have patients that would qualify for the study? How many? If it is a trial for hypertension, what percentage of your hypertension patients would qualify? The same question should be raised for a trial in any therapeutic specialty. If the percentage of your patients that would be excluded is high, then it is going to be very difficult to fill the study.

You need to accurately assess the limitations of your own patient database. The exclusion criteria may be realistic. But how many patients do you have that fall into the general therapeutic category? For example, if the protocol is for a drug to treat acute back strain, how many patients came to your office during the past year with that complaint? If an investigator lacks patients that fit the criteria, then the only way to fill the study will be through advertising and referrals from other physicians. Although studies can be filled in that manner, it presents a challenge that the novice site would be wise to avoid.

After assessing whether the inclusion-exclusion criteria are realistic, a site needs to evaluate whether the protocol demands too much of the patients. A site may have a number of patients that are eligible for the study, but will patients stay in the study? To evaluate this question, you need to carefully review the Schedule of Events in the protocol. This part of the protocol precisely describes the procedures and tests that may be performed and what will be required of the patient. Although patients are reimbursed for their time, a protocol that is particularly demanding of patients – both in terms of time and the procedures that are involved – will scare patients away. Even if they agree to volunteer, the dropout rate is likely to be high.

For example, if a trial for hypertension requires a patient to wear a 24-hour blood pressure monitoring device several times during a six-month study, many patients will refuse to participate for that reason alone. This is particularly true if they have ever had to wear one before and have been awakened throughout the night by the inflation of the cuff. Or consider a study that requires a patient to remain in the physician's office for up to six hours on a single visit. How many people will volunteer for a study that requires that much of their time? Here is a simple rule of thumb: the more a study requires of the patient, the greater the number of dropouts during the course of a study. A sponsor is going to evaluate a site's performance based on the number of patients it can retain throughout the study. Ultimately, this is what the sponsor is paying for: patients who can be evaluated. In fact, an effective measurement of a site's performance is the ratio of number of patients entered to the number of patients completed.

 ## Creativity Counts

An investigator in a trial has agreed to follow the protocol without deviating from it in any manner. At times, I believe that a successful investigator enrolls his or her study despite the protocol. This means that a certain amount of creativity comes into play. This can be a challenge, and, believe it or not, a lot of fun. For example, in studies for acute exacerbation of chronic bronchitis, frequently the factor that hinders patient enrollment is obtaining a sputum that will grow pathogens. For most patients, it is very difficult to produce a sample on command, particularly if it is late in the day. Our solution was to mail all of our chronic bronchitis patients a sputum bottle decorated with red ribbons. We requested that they keep the bottles beside their beds, and that whenever they were scheduled for office visits, that they put their first morning sputum in the bottles, and bring the bottles with them.

As you evaluate a protocol, you also need to assess what impact the trial will have on your time and on your regular practice. A study that requires every patient to be seen at no later than 8 a.m. may be a problem if the physician is regularly in surgery at that hour. A study that requires a patient to be seen 72 hours after initial enrollment may be impossible for you to do, if you have office hours at that particular location only twice a week.

As part of this self-assessment, a site should carefully analyze the protocol to identify every single procedure, laboratory test, and event that will have to be performed. Can your site successfully perform these procedures or successfully farm them out to suppliers? A site needs to determine precisely what will be required and evaluate whether it has the resources to accomplish these tasks.

In summary, the smart investigative site will reject protocols that have unrealistic inclusion-exclusion criteria or are unnecessarily demanding. The smart site will also reject protocols that aren't compatible with its own capabilities and regular practice routines. For research sites, analyzing protocols is one of the keys to success.

Negotiating the Budget

There are few topics in clinical research that will engender spirited discussions as quickly as budgeting. The process can be time-consuming, confusing and maddening. And, of course, a site's skill in preparing a budget is critical to making clinical research a profitable enterprise. It is easy for even an experienced site to lose money on a study.

Traditionally, sponsors have asked investigative sites to prepare line-item budgets. As part of the protocol, the sponsor outlines a Schedule of Events that is supposed to serve as a guide to investigators as they construct their budgets. The investigative site itemizes a fee for each item and then tallies the fees for an overall budget. The theory behind this process is that the site is being reimbursed on a fee-for-service basis for everything it does and usually at a higher rate than is standard in general practice.

Most budgets are still prepared this way. However, a few sponsors and CROs are now presenting candidate sites with take-it-or-leave-it per-patient budgets. It doesn't matter what the site calculates it will need to be reasonably reimbursed. The site is simply asked: will it do the study for this fixed per-patient fee? This budget may allow for some billing for extraordinary costs, but, in general, it is a bottom-line approach that is much less flexible than the traditional method.

In either instance, the site needs to pay attention to potential hidden-cost traps that can turn what appears to be a high-profit trial into a money drain. In clinical research, a site needs to anticipate that the time and effort necessary to successfully complete a study will be significantly greater than it would be to treat a similar number of regular-practice patients. It must negotiate a budget that provides adequate reimbursement for that extra time and effort.

The Financial Squeeze

The economics of research have changed dramatically during the past 10 years. A decade ago, pharmaceutical companies basically had to court academic physicians with their grant proposals. Physicians at academic medical centers were often even reluctant to take the grants. As a result, pharmaceutical companies were typically very generous with their grants. They needed the academic physicians both for their ability to conduct their trials and for their "thought leader" prestige. The pharmaceutical companies wanted the prestige of academic physicians to help sell their drugs after they were approved. In this environment, there was little market pressure curbing research fees.

Today, pharmaceutical companies are much more cost conscious. There are two factors that are driving this change. The first is simple supply and demand. The number of investigators has risen so dramatically that pharmaceutical companies can now quickly gather a pool of candidate investigators that is much larger than the number they need for a study. They can then use this competition to help keep their costs down. Although pharmaceutical companies won't select the sites solely on the basis of cost, they do now consider cost as part of the selection criteria. The increased competition also has resulted in some sites being willing to accept low-ball budgets, a market pressure that reduces grant size.

The second factor is a database called PICAS. In the late 1980s, a number of large pharmaceutical companies agreed to provide the company DataEdge with their data, detailing what they spent on investigator grants. The data included information on fees for particular laboratory tests and itemized fees for physician services. The pharmaceutical companies now use the PICAS database to determine average fees paid to investigators and base their grants on this database. Although a few pharmaceutical companies may try to select sites that accept grants below the norm, most major ones will simply try to keep the average per-patient fees for a study, across all sites, at close to the PICAS norm. The PICAS database provides sponsors with a tool to keep their investigator costs down.

There is some question about the accuracy of this database. If PICAS uses a particular methodology for the calculation of a fee, it may vary greatly from the methodology used at your site. For example, if you need a mammography as part of the trial, your institution might require that it be broken down into a technical and a mechanical component with a charge for each of these. PICAS may have calculated this cost as a single combined charge that is much less than the two charges you have to consider. Of course, PICAS also occasionally overestimates costs as well. Ultimately, as long as the overall budget is in the range you require, you should not worry too much about the individual components. I say this with a bit of caution because if certain visits or procedures need to be repeated, a site can find itself reimbursed at a lower level than what is necessary to cover its costs.

Grants are lower than they used to be, but not so low that a research site can't turn an excellent profit. Even with these price pressures, the well-run site can still generate profit margins of 25% and above. In fact, it is not unusual for a well-run site to be profitable to the tune of 40% after all expenses including contracted labor are paid. The physician or physician group who incorporates clinical research into a general practice can still do very well. But because the market isn't as generous as it was 10 years ago, the investigator has to be more skilled at negotiating "smart" budgets.

Preparing a Budget

Research grants do reimburse physicians at a higher level than is standard for normal practice. This is necessary because of the extra time and effort involved. Considerable time is spent in negotiating study contracts, fulfilling regulatory requirements related to conducting clinical research, recruiting patients, filling out case report forms, and interacting with the monitors and sponsor throughout the course of the study. The pharmaceutical companies recognize that extra time and effort is required and will generally negotiate budgets that pay for this extra effort.

One way to prepare a budget, which some experienced investigators say works for them, is simply to ask the sponsor what it expects to pay, on a per-patient basis. Those who use this approach say that, in most instances, the pharmaceutical company will give an honest answer. Often, the investigator will find that the sponsor is expecting to pay a higher amount than the site would have asked for on its own. Also, a site that has a reputation for quality and delivering patients can probably submit a budget that is 15% higher than the sponsor's target fee and still get the grant. Obviously, a novice investigator will need to submit a budget that is in line with the norm.

The smart site is also going to do its own budget analysis. There are market pressures keeping grants down, and pharmaceutical companies are taking advantage of this new economic environment. A site needs to develop a skill in analyzing budgets both to negotiate profitable budgets and to know when to turn down studies. Turning down studies can be an essential aspect of operating a site profitably.

The first step in constructing a proposed budget is to assign fees for each step in the schedule of events. Here is a sample schedule of events for an eight-week hypertensive trial that involves four patient visits.

Study visit	1	2	3	4
Study week	2	4	6	8
Informed consent	X			
Medical history	X			
Physical examination	X			
Vital signs	X	X	X	X
Electrocardiogram	X	X		
Fasting blood draw	X	X		
Pregnancy screen	X			
24-hour blood pressure monitor		X	X	
Dispense medications		X	X	
Adverse event assessment		X	X	X

First, calculate patient-visit fees:

Visit one

Medical history:	This is to be done by the physician-investigator.	$100
Medical physical:	This is also done by the investigator or a subinvestigator.	$100
Coordinator time:	The coordinator can take vital signs, secure the informed consent, etc.	$75
Electrocardiogram:		$100
Blood draw:	This is based on a protocol requiring the blood sample to be shipped to a central laboratory. If the site sends the blood draw to its own laboratory, it must add a laboratory fee.	$25
Pregnancy screen:	This assumes a urine pregnancy test done in the office with testing material supplied by the sponsor.	$25
Additional charges:	Office visit:	$75
	Secretarial charge for visit:	$25
	Patient stipend:	$25

Total charges for visit one $550

Visit two

Coordinator	$75
Visit	$75
Secretary	$25
24-hour blood pressure monitor	The monitor will be supplied by the sponsor. The $150 charge reflects the time it will take the coordinator to apply the instrument and to record and transmit the data generated by the monitor. — $200
Patient stipend	The higher stipend for this visit is due to the requirement that the patient wear the monitor, which is uncomfortable, for 24 hours. — $100

Total charges for visit two $475

Visit three

The requirements for visit three are the same as for visit two.
Total charges for visit three $475

Visit four

Physical	$100
Electrocardiogram	$100
Blood draw	$25

Coordinator $75
Office visit $75
Secretary $25
Patient stipend $25
Total charges for visit four **$425**

Total per-patient fees for the four-visit study:

Visit one $550
Visit two $475
Visit three $475
Visit four $425
Total **$1925**

Overhead

A site also needs to be reimbursed for its study start-up costs. By some estimates, 25% of the time spent on a study is for initiating the study: negotiating the budget, signing the contract and securing approval from an institutional review board. At the very least, a site should seek to negotiate an overhead fee of 15% to cover study start-up expenses.

Some pharmaceutical companies will only pay overhead fees to hospitals or teaching facilities. If that is the case, a site may need to increase its per-patient visit fees by 15% in order to cover study start-up expenses and the additional time and labor associated with responding to inquiries from the monitor during the course of the study and after the study is completed.

Other Routine Fees

In order to conduct a trial, a site must get approval from an IRB. In some studies, a sponsor will hire a central IRB to provide this review process for all the nonacademic sites. In that case, the site does not need to budget a separate IRB fee because it will be paid directly by the sponsor. But if the site needs to obtain approval from a local IRB, then this expense must be included in the budget. Do not forget that most IRBs charge additional fees for approvals of amendments and a fee to maintain the IRB's supervision of the trial. Make sure that these items are left open because additional charges may be passed on to the sponsor for reimbursement.

Sponsors are often willing to pay for an advertising budget. They want sites to recruit patients as quickly as possible, and they will reimburse sites that want to place radio and newspaper ads. For a site seeking to enroll 16 patients in an eight-week hypertension study, a typical advertising allowance might be about $1,200. This is a separate budget item.

Estimating Number of Patients

The final step in the budgeting process is estimating how many patients you can expect to enroll. This can be tricky.

Because sponsors place such importance on patient recruitment, many sites are tempted to exaggerate their capabilities during the site-selection process. In order to secure grants, investigators may provide very optimistic estimates of the number of patients they believe they can enroll into the study. Although being overly optimistic may help a site to win an initial grant, it can backfire in the long run. At the end of a study, a site will be judged more on whether it fully enrolled its trial (in other words, enrolled the number of patients it promised to enroll), rather than on the absolute number of patients it enrolled. A site that has contracted to enroll 10 patients and enrolls 10 will be viewed as successfully meeting its estimates; a site that has a contract to enroll 30 patients and enrolls 15 will be viewed as having fallen short. This means that the site has to walk a fine line between estimating a number of patients that will keep the sponsors and CROs interested and what the site can actually produce.

In most instances, being slightly conservative won't put an absolute cap on your budget either. Studies are routinely delayed because of poor patient recruitment. A site that has met its budget quota early can almost always get permission from the sponsor to enroll additional patients. The site that meets its patient-enrollment estimates and then exceeds its quota develops an excellent reputation. This is the kind of reputation that can help make a site's business opportunities soar. Actually, the additional patients entered into a trial are frequently those who produce the highest net profit. This is because the system is already in place, and your staff is trained for this particular trial. The extra patient allocation is found money.

Proposed Budget for Hypertension Study

Once you have estimated the number of patients that you can expect to enroll, you will need to multiply this number by your per-patient fee to establish a base amount. For the hypertension trial described above, this base amount would be calculated as follows:

$1,900 per patient x 16 ....$30,400
15% overhead $4,560
IRB $1,500

Advertising allowance $1,200
Total **$37,660**

This budget would provide a site with approximately $2,000 in fees for each patient retained through the four visits. Since this is a simple study, this budget would provide a site with a good profit margin. Even so, the budget preparation is not yet finished.

Hidden Costs

One of the biggest complaints that sites have about research budgets is that they don't account for hidden costs. A site that doesn't adequately prepare for hidden costs can easily lose money on a trial.

First, the schedule of events has been prepared by the sponsor. It is easy for the sponsor to overlook tasks that will be required by the protocol. For example, a protocol may require telephone visits. The coordinator will be required to periodically call the patients during the study. But this function may not be sharply detailed in the schedule of events, and thus easy to miss as a site prepares its budget. The site will need to charge for the coordinator's time.

Second, during the course of a trial, the sponsor or CRO is likely to make additional requests of a site that aren't covered in the protocol. Perhaps the site will be asked to add an additional page to a case report form. Or perhaps a protocol amendment will require an additional office visit for each patient. Although a site can't put a fee into its budget for these contingency items, it can negotiate a clause in the contract stating that if they occur, the sponsor will pay for them.

Third, sites regularly underestimate the time and expense associated with screening costs. How many people will need to be screened to find an eligible patient? The more strict the eligibility criteria, the greater the number of people who will have to be screened. Screening visits are real costs. A site needs to analyze the protocol in order to anticipate this screening expense and try to get some compensation for it.

The full extent of this screening expense may not show up during the trial. Consider a trial for a new oral hypoglycemic agent. One of the inclusion criteria might be that the patient has a hemoglobin A1C of 7% to 8% at visit three (after having been off all medications and on a normal diet for four weeks). Perhaps 25% of the patients who enroll into the study will survive this restriction. This means that a site may have to perform as many as 12 patient visits to get one subject through visit three. In order to make the trial worthwhile, a site will need to get paid for all 12 visits.

At times, despite a site's best budgeting efforts, it finds that it has made mistakes in its budget and is losing money on the study. If so, a site can approach the monitor and request an increase in fees. Often, the sponsor will adjust the site's budget, if the request appears justified.

In most instances, the sponsor won't even let a site begin the study if its budget is too far below the norm. An unusually low budget is a signal that the site hasn't done an adequate job of analyzing the protocol (and thus doesn't realize what will be involved), or the site is so inexperienced at clinical research that it can't anticipate the extra time and effort involved in conducting a clinical trial. Although there are cost pressures present in the industry, sponsors still want to nurture a sense of fair play in their interactions with physicians conducting research for them.

The novice investigator may find constructing a budget daunting. The best advice for the novice investigator may be to simply trust the sponsor. Ask the sponsor what it expects to pay, and, unless it seems unreasonable, agree to conduct the study for that amount. In this way, you can still make the leap into clinical research, without worrying about the intricacies of constructing a budget. Preparing budgets is an art that is developed with experience.

The Contract

Every sponsor and CRO with whom you work will have its own standard contract. A novice investigator should always have an initial contract reviewed by an attorney. Once a site gains experience, signing a contract is usually easily accomplished. In many instances, companies now ask whether a contract is necessary.

Academic physicians will typically need to negotiate contracts that include clauses relating to the right to publish and other academic integrity issues. For the private-practice physician, there are two primary concerns with the contract. First, you should always ask for indemnification. There is some question about the effectiveness of indemnification, but it is still worthwhile to insist that it be present in the contract.

Second, you should carefully review the payment schedule outlined in the contract. As discussed earlier, payments in the clinical research industry can lag many, many months behind. The contract will stipulate the amount of the up-front payment and the study milestones that will trigger interim payments. In order to minimize the cash flow problem, you can try to negotiate a larger up-front payment, or a steady schedule of interim payments. Although you may not be able to press too hard on this issue without stirring up resistance, at least you should be aware of the slow payment schedules and prepare for it.

Other less important issues include the right to publish, ownership of new discoveries and things such as the retention of records. The financial contract is always separate from the agreement to function as a clinical investigator. Financial agreements are private, and neither the IRB nor the

FDA has a right to review them. Consequently these should be stored in a different place than all the regulatory documents. Keep the agreements private and do not allow them to be reviewed by anyone other than your associates and accountant.

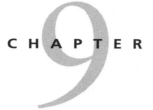

CHAPTER

Regulatory Requirements

- Filing a 1572 Form
- The Investigator's Meeting

Once a site has negotiated the budget and signed the contract, it will need to complete several regulatory steps before it can begin conducting the study. All clinical trials in the United States are conducted under the supervision of two separate and very different types of organizations: the Food and Drug Administration (FDA) and the institutional review board (IRB) that has jurisdiction over each clinical trial.

Filing a 1572 Form

The principal investigator listed on the grant must complete a 1572 form that the sponsor will file with the FDA. The 1572 form provides the FDA with the investigator's name, address and CV. The investigator must list the names of all sub-investigators who will be assisting in the research as well as each location where the trial will be carried out. A copy of the protocol is attached to the form as well. A copy of the 1572 form is appended to this book.

On the back of the 1572 is a set of statements to which the investigator agrees by his or her signature on this form. It is important to recognize what you are committing yourself to by your signature.

1. You, as an investigator, agree to conduct the trial according to the protocol and not to change the protocol except when a patient's safety is at stake.
2. You agree to personally conduct the trial. You must be hands-on.
3. You agree to inform your patients that they are participating in a clinical trial, and you agree to get proper consent.
4. You, as an investigator, agree to properly report any adverse event.
5. You certify that you have read and understand the investigator brochure or manual and are aware of any potential side effect caused by this substance.
6. You agree to be responsible for those working under your supervision on this trial.
7. You agree to keep accurate records and to make them available for inspection.
8. You agree to work under the direction of a qualified IRB and to promptly report any unanticipated problems or events to this board. Also, you agree not to make any changes in the protocol without notifying the IRB of those changes in advance.
9. Finally, you agree to comply with all other requirements regarding the obligations of a clinical investigator in regulations 21 CFR Part 312.

In short, the 1572 form is a contract in which the investigator promises the FDA that he or she will conduct the trial in accordance with Good Clinical Practices. It is vital that you as an investigator understand each of these points.

It is important to take this form seriously. You need to read it closely and to fill it out accurately. For example, if an investigator states that the study will be conducted a specific location, it is not legal to enroll patients from another location unless that second location is listed on the 1572 form. In a similar vein, any physician who will help you treat study patients must be listed as a sub-investigator. A resident coming to an investigator's office two or three nights a week cannot see study patients unless he or she is listed on this form.

Historically, many of the modern regulations governing clinical research in the United States are the result of the thalidomide tragedy that occurred in the 1960s. The United States was spared the brunt of the effects of this drug, but there was still enough exposure to stimulate a close look at the laws surrounding human research. The result was the Kefauver-Harris amendment of 1962. This legislation required that drug manufacturers prove effectiveness and safety before marketing any new product. Additional legislation was included regarding consenting human subjects and reporting of adverse effects. Also, the FDA was placed in a supervisory position. Since then there have been several modifications of laws governing research.

The patient protection law is consolidated in the Code of Federal Regulations under section 21 CFR part 50, appended to this book. These regulations address the appropriate treatment of subjects in human trials and the laws that govern their treatment. It is important that any clinical investigator be familiar with them as well as with such documents as the Helsinki accords.

At this time, it is appropriate to review all the statements to which you agreed, on the 1572, in light of these laws. The first is "you, as an investigator, agree to conduct the trial according to the protocol and not to change the protocol except when a patient's safety is at stake." This statement addresses two issues. The first is that clinical research is not the practice of medicine. When you do a trial, the protocol comes first, and the physician has no ability to modify or stretch the limits of this document. The first purpose of research is to collect data, not to treat the patient. Therefore, the protocol is the priority. The second issue is that despite what the study states, you as a physician may do no harm to that patient. This means that if potential harm could occur to a patient because of his or her participation in a trial, that patient should be removed from the trial and his or her treatment should be prioritized.

The second statement is "you agree to personally conduct the trial. You must be hands-on." This statement means that you are personally responsible for the conduct of the trial. It may not be delegated to a resident or an intern or an investigator at another site. Clinical trials require your personal supervision.

The third statement deals with informed consent. It states "you agree to inform your patients that they are participating in a clinical trial and you agree to get proper consent." The elements of informed consent are delineated in section 50.25 of these federal regulations. It is worth reviewing them here.

1. A statement that the study involves research, an explanation of the purpose of the research and the expected duration of the subject's participation, a description of the procedures to be followed, and identification of any procedures that are experimental.
2. A description of any reasonably foreseeable risk or discomforts to the subject.
3. A description of any benefits to the subject or to others that may be reasonably expected from the research.
4. A disclosure of appropriate alternative procedures or course of treatment, if any, that might be advantageous to the subject.
5. A statement describing the extent, if any, to which confidentiality of records identifying the subject will be maintained and that notes the possibility that the FDA may inspect the records.

6. For research involving more than the minimal risk, an explanation of whether any medical treatments are available if injury occurs and, if so, what they consist of, or where further information may be obtained.
7. An explanation of whom to contact for answers to pertinent questions about research subjects' rights, and whom to contact in the event of research-related injury to the subject.
8. A statement that participation is voluntary, that refusal to participate will involve no loss of benefits to which the subject is otherwise entitled, and that the subject may discontinue participation at any time without penalty or loss of benefits to which the subject is otherwise entitled.

There are additional elements of consent that may be appropriate to particular trials. These are also delineated in 50.25 and can be found in the appendix of this book.

If the sponsor of a trial is using a central IRB, the sponsor will supply a consent form that can easily be modified for use by every site. Each site will simply have to alter the template to include specific site information such as address and emergency telephone number. The central IRB will then be asked to approve the consent form specifically for your site. The IRB will pay attention to your CV to make certain that you are qualified to function as an investigator. A medical degree goes a long way toward verifying your qualifications, as does any specialty training involving the therapeutic arena in which the trial is to take place.

If the sponsor does not provide a master consent form, then it is the responsibility of the investigator to create one that is in accordance with federal regulations. (Again, FDA regulation 21 CFR 50 details the requirements for a consent form; a sample consent form is in the appendix of this book.) An essential requirement is that the form be written in easy-to-understand language that does not require a medical background. The form should be written at the sixth-grade reading level. Also, if the patient speaks only Spanish, for example, the consent must be in Spanish. It is essential that all of the elements specified in the FDA regulations are included in the consent form.

One way to create a consent form is to find an existing form for the general therapeutic category and then modify it for the study at hand. A novice investigator can ask the sponsor for a sample consent form. To modify a consent form, the investigator will have to change the title, protocol number, date, description of the drug, and the description of the trial's objective. Every consent form needs to include these additional items as specified by 50.25 of the federal code as alluded to above.

- A description of the investigational drug and the objective of the trial. This section must include a side-effect profile of the drug (which can be found in the protocol). It is customary to add a general disclaimer that not all side effects are known. If the protocol calls for comparing the investigational drug to a standard treatment, the side effects for the standard treatment must be described as well. This information can be found in the Physicians' Desk Reference or in a package insert. This section should also include information on the total number of patients and sites that will be involved in the study.

- A description of the protocol and what will be required of the patient. This section must inform the patient of the number of visits and the various procedures that will be required. The patient should be informed of the right to drop out of the study at any time. The stipend that will be paid to the patient should be clearly detailed. Please note: A stipend must not be used in a coercive manner. It is inappropriate to withhold the entire stipend if a patient does not complete the study. A stipend should be parcelled out on a per-visit basis. However, it is considered appropriate to give the patient a bonus for completing the final visit.
- A description of the risks involved in the trial. The patient must be told of all risks associated with taking the investigational therapy. For example, if the trial is for a hypertension drug, the patients must be informed they will have to stop taking their current blood pressure medications, and that this may lead to a rise in their blood pressure. In all trials, the patients must also be informed of any alternative therapies that may be available for the particular disease or condition being studied, and that they do not have to participate in the trial to receive appropriate medical care.
- A description of their rights as a study volunteer. The patient must be informed of a contact at the IRB who can answer questions regarding the study or a patient's rights as a research subject. The patient also must be promised that if significant new information becomes known that might affect a patient's willingness to participate in the study, the physician will inform the volunteer of this information.
- All other requirements are described in regulation 21 CRF 50. (See sample consent form in the appendix.)

There are also specific requirements for obtaining consent. First, consent should be administered by the investigator or sub investigator. Second, there should be a specific statement written by the investigator in the patient's medical record that all questions were reviewed and answered. This needs to be signed and dated by the investigator. Also, the consent form needs to be witnessed. The best individual to do this is a relative of the patient, if one is present. Otherwise, a coordinator or a receptionist will do. A copy of the consent form needs to be given to the patient, and the fact that this has been done also needs to be recorded in the source document (patient's records).

To return to the statements on the 1572 form, the fourth statement is "you, as an investigator, agree to properly report any adverse event." This is an essential responsibility for an investigator and an area where mistakes are frequently made. Any serious unexpected adverse event needs to be reported to the sponsoring company and to the IRB within 24 hours. The sponsoring company is then required to report these events to the FDA within three days. "Unexpected" means events that are not alluded to in the drug manual or that are new. All serious adverse events, expected or not, must be reported by the investigator to both the IRB and the sponsor within 10 days.

A serious adverse event is one that suggests that a significant hazard has occurred to the patient. The event can be fatal or life-threatening, including those that cause permanent disabilities or inpatient hospitalization. Any event associated with an overdose, a death, a congenital anomaly or cancer is always considered serious.

It is of utmost importance that an investigator leave a "paper trail" when reporting adverse events. Document to whom you report, when you report and the outcome of the conversation. It is particularly important when you make phone contact with the IRB and the sponsoring company. This also applies each and every time anyone from your site speaks to any individual at the sponsoring company, the CRO, the IRB or the patient. Document everything. Keep meticulous phone logs of all conversations. It is really quite easy to do this. It simply requires that you and your employees develop the right habits.

The next element you have agreed to on the back of the 1572 is the fifth. It states "you certify that you have read and understand the investigator brochure or manual and are aware of any potential side effect caused by this substance." This requires little explanation. You must read and understand the drug, the comparative agent and the protocol. This is truly a reasonable and essential request.

The sixth item on the 1572 states "you agree to be responsible for those working under your supervision on this trial." This clearly delineates that the main responsibility is yours as the investigator. You should not depend on individuals at a CRO or an SMO to assume your responsibility even if they agree to. The investigator is responsible for reporting adverse events, and even though a well-intentioned monitor from a CRO might tell you not to worry, that he or she would take care of reporting a particular event to the sponsor, do it yourself anyway. Always err on the side of over-reporting. It is better that a sponsor hears about a serious adverse event from two sources than not at all.

Also, this statement means that actions taken by your staff and coordinators are clearly your responsibility, so make sure you know what is going on. It is a good idea to have weekly staff meetings with all those individuals at your site who are involved in a particular protocol. Make sure that all problems relevant to that protocol are put on the table and that "action items" are decided on to resolve them. You, as an investigator, must be intimately involved and must have full knowledge of the conduct of the trial.

The seventh item on the back of the 1572 states "you agree to keep accurate records and to make them available for inspection." It is also necessary to make your records available to the IRB and to the sponsor for inspection. Accurate records do not just include the case report forms. The most significant part of keeping accurate records are the source documents. These are the backbone of clinical research. Source documents are those records and files that support the information extracted in the case report forms.

These consist of the patient's medical records, the office appointment book, telephone logs and all the other notes.

When you do a clinical trial, it is essential that a record be maintained that can be looked at by an auditor and that the history of interactions during that trial period be clearly and obviously apparent. A paper trail must always be left. Each piece of that trail must support all the other pieces. There must be no contradictions. If the date for a visit is on the case report forms as July 14, it also should be July 14 on the patient records and in the office appointment book. If the blood pressure in the case report form is recorded as 145/90, the same must be true in the patient records.

All notes in the patient records should be dated and signed by those entering them. It should be clear exactly who is recording what. This is not complicated to do. It merely requires that good habits and standard operating procedures be established. Every time anyone in the office has any conversation or interaction involving a particular trial, it needs to be recorded, signed and dated. This includes all phone conversations and all discussions with patients. In fact, an essential element of source documentation is a screening log. On this log should be recorded every patient approached by the staff to enter the trial whether they agree or not to enter the trial.

Finally, it is important that these source documents be legible, so take your time. It only takes a few seconds to do these things properly.

The eighth element to which an investigator agrees by signing the 1572 is "you agree to work under the direction of a qualified IRB and to promptly report any unanticipated problems or event to this board. Also, you agree not to make any changes in the protocol without notifying the IRB of those changes in advance."

As I've stated before, the investigator also must obtain approval from an IRB to conduct the study. The IRB will review the protocol and the informed consent form to be signed by patients. During the course of the study, the investigator must inform the IRB of all serious adverse events, and of all protocol amendments. The IRB must also approve any patient-recruitment advertisements.

The FDA mandates that an IRB have at least five members, including representation from both sexes and at least one person who has a nonscientific background. The IRB is charged with reviewing the protocol to ensure that it has a valid scientific objective, and that it does not pose unnecessary risks to the patients. Although the IRB is charged with guarding the welfare of the patient, the IRB also provides a safety net for the investigators. IRB oversight helps investigators conduct research in a moral, ethical manner.

It is becoming common for a sponsor to contract with a commercial IRB to provide this review for all of its sites conducting a particular protocol. The use of a central IRB can greatly relieve the individual site of this regulatory burden. The central IRB will approve the protocol and a patient consent form to be used by all sites. The individual site will simply need to get the central IRB to approve any advertisements it may want to use during the course of the study.

If an investigator is conducting research at an academic medical center or a hospital, it is likely that the institution will have its own IRB. This can prove to be a barrier for an investigator. Many institutional IRBs meet only once a month, which can make getting IRB review a very slow process. Because sponsors want sites to start their studies quickly, they may avoid selecting investigators who have to petition institutional IRBs. Also, hospital IRBs often include members who are not particularly familiar with the requirements and regulations surrounding research. This lack of familiarity can cause the IRB to raise objections to a protocol that an experienced IRB would never raise. All the other sites in a study will be busy enrolling patients, while the hospital-based site is still trying to obtain an IRB review.

An investigator who must use a hospital or medical school IRB can do several things to make this process go smoothly. One approach is to request that the institution's IRB waive its supervision for a particular protocol and allow the trial to proceed under the supervision of the commercial IRB. Another is for the investigator to become familiar with the institution's IRB and to submit the protocol in a format that the IRB will find easy to review. Finally, the investigator should personally present the protocol at the IRB meeting. By attending the meeting, the investigator can answer any questions the IRB may have and can clear up any misconceptions the board may have about the protocol. And, as you might expect, an IRB is much less likely to turn down a protocol when the investigator is present. There is one other advantage to working with a commercial IRB. The commercial IRBs generally provide closer oversight during the course of a trial, and this can help prevent the investigator from making mistakes and missing required updates. For example, an investigator may be required to update the IRB on the progress of the study every six months and to notify the IRB when the trial is completed. A commercial IRB will send investigators written reminders to supply these updates.

It typically costs $1,000 to $2,500 to use a commercial IRB for a study. The IRB will also charge for additional services such as approving amendments and advertisements. If the sponsor has hired a central IRB for a study, it will pay these costs. If not, the investigative site must include this expense in its budget.

An IRB also has ongoing oversight of a clinical trial, and it is required that an investigator give the IRB periodic updates on the process of the trial as well as immediate updates on any serious adverse events. An investigator cannot change anything about a trial without IRB approval. A site may not add physical locations to the trial, add sub-investigators, or change any of the protocol procedures without having an amendment approved by the IRB. This is one of the areas where the FDA has identified many investigator errors occurring. Investigators neglect to inform their IRB of these issues, and it is a clear violation of an investigator's agreement as stated on the 1572 form.

Also an IRB must review and sign off on any advertisements that will be viewed by potential subjects. All ads must be approved for wording, intent and other components by your IRB. Again, this is something that is frequently overlooked by the investigator.

The final element agreed to, by the investigator, when he or she signs the 1572 is "you agree to comply with all other requirements regarding the obligations of a clinical investigator in regulations 21 CFR Part 312." Take a look at these regulations in their entirety. They are appended to this book.

The Investigators' Meeting

Once all the sites have been selected, the sponsor or CRO managing the project will hold an investigators' meeting. The principal investigator and lead study coordinator from each site are expected to attend. These meetings are usually a mix of business and pleasure. The investigator and coordinator will have an opportunity to raise questions about the study, meet new people (an important marketing opportunity) and enjoy a mini-vacation.

It is essential that an investigator attends and brings a study coordinator to the meeting. An investigator who does not bother to attend these meetings will be perceived as uninterested in the trial. The study coordinator needs to be present as well so that he or she can be well versed in all of the minute details of the protocol and regulatory requirements. The sponsor or CRO will chalk up two strikes against a site that doesn't have a coordinator present at the meeting either. Many investigators, by way of providing extra incentive to their coordinators, pay them time and a half for their travel time and meeting time.

An investigators' meeting usually lasts one or two days. The actual sessions typically take six to 10 hours. For the investigator, the most important session is the discussion of the protocol. The protocol is reviewed, and all the investigators are supposed to come to a uniform understanding of how the protocol is to be implemented. Investigators are also given an opportunity to comment on the protocol's logic and feasibility. A sponsor will often amend the protocol, including inclusion and exclusion criteria, in response to the investigators' comments and criticisms.

Many investigators are surprised by what they hear during the protocol-review session. They often haven't read the protocol in full detail and suddenly are voicing objections to all the work that is involved. They complain that the study is more complex and demanding than they realized and that their budgets are too low. To which the sponsor and CRO are apt to reply: Didn't you read the protocol before preparing your budgets? As such, the review session is a good check on a site's study start-up procedures. If the investigator and study coordinator are constantly surprised by what they hear, then their site is not doing an adequate job of assessing the protocol before agreeing to conduct the study.

Most of the other sessions during the one or two days are more important to the coordinator than to the investigator. However, by attending the sessions, the investigator will get a better feel for the amount of work involved in the study and the logistical demands that will be placed on the coordinator. There is also always a session devoted to regulatory issues. For the novice investigator, these sessions can provide important information. However, for a seasoned investigator, they can be a challenge to sit through because all regulatory sessions address basically the same issues.

The investigators' meeting also provides a site with an important marketing opportunity. This meeting may be the only opportunity for an investigator to actually meet the sponsor's or CRO's project manager. You can use this opportunity to inform the project manager of your interest in conducting other protocols. Often, the sponsor or CRO will be actively seeking investigators for protocols in other therapeutic areas, and you can inform them of your site's capability to conduct this research. And even if the people at the meeting are not managing the other protocols, you can get contact information from them.

The meeting also presents an opportunity to exchange leads about study opportunities with the other investigators. It's a give-and-take deal. By sharing what you know about other study opportunities, you can expect to gather leads from the other investigators. A common rule of thumb is that every investigators' meeting should provide leads that eventually result in at least one new grant. This is a good way for an investigator to build his or her research business.

In general, the meetings are a pleasure to attend. The sponsor often uses a start-up meeting as a way to provide an extra reward, or incentive, to the sites. The meetings are usually held in cities attractive to tourists, at top resorts and hotels. Orlando and Phoenix are common locations in the winter. They are also usually scheduled at the end of the week, making it possible for the investigators and study coordinators to extend their stay to create a small vacation. Often, the sponsor will pay the investigator and coordinator a small stipend as well.

Finally, an investigator can use the meeting to collect continuing education credits. Usually, all an investigator will need to do is submit the agenda to an accreditation board.

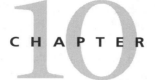

CHAPTER

Conducting The Study

- Good Clinical Practices
- The Study Binder
- Securing Informed Consent
- Source Documents
- Case Report Form
- Reporting Adverse Events
- Standard Operating Procedures (SOPs)
- Other Study Conduct Tips

The investigators' meeting is over. The protocol has been reviewed, the budget negotiated and the contract signed. Now you are ready to actually conduct the trial. This will require following Good Clinical Practice regulations and meticulously recording all patient data.

Good Clinical Practices

Good Clinical Practice, in reality, is more a nonspecific term that is applied by those in government and in the pharmaceutical industry to a group of related regulations that define the responsibility of individuals involved in the clinical research process. These regulations apply to the sponsor and its employees, the IRB, and the investigator and those who work at the site. Of course, the CROs function as surrogate sponsors and are also subject to these regulations.

The Good Clinical Practices that govern clinical research are based on FDA regulations. These regulations include the 1987 IND Rewrite regulations that define the responsibilities of the investigator. Many of these practices relating to study start-up practices have been discussed, or alluded to, in earlier chapters. Once a study is underway, Good Clinical Practices require the investigator to:

- Obtain informed consent from every study volunteer.
- Maintain accurate case histories for all study subjects.
- Maintain accurate records detailing the receipt, dispensation and final disposition of the study drug.
- Notify the IRB of all amendments to the study protocol.
- Report all adverse events to the sponsor, and immediately report all "serious and unexpected" adverse events to the sponsor and IRB.
- Maintain a record of accreditation for all laboratories used during the study.
- Retain all records related to the trial for at least two years following the FDA's review of the sponsor's New Drug Application, or following the sponsor's notification of the FDA that the development of the drug has been discontinued.

Good Clinical Practice guidelines carry the authority of law. The FDA can – and will – institute legal action against any investigator who violates the guidelines. Sanctions include limiting the investigator's ability to conduct research and placing the investigator on a "blacklist" that prohibits the investigator from conducting any research.

The Study Binder

In clinical research, investigators are required to compile a detailed regulatory file. The study binder is a tool for making sure that all necessary documents are collected. Normally, the sponsoring organization provides this binder to each site. The site is required to include all the elements and to continually fill this binder as a trial progresses. The study binder will have designated sections for organizing all the required regulatory papers. The papers to be filed in the study binder include:

- A signed, original copy of the protocol and all amendments. (Not a photocopy).
- An original 1572 form.
- Updated copies of CVs for the investigator and sub-investigators. These should be signed and dated.

- Copies of laboratory certifications and reference ranges for laboratory values.
- Copies of the drug brochure and, when indicated, package inserts.
- Letter of approval from the IRB.
- The original signed and stamped IRB-approved consent form.
- Any advertisements used in the study with the IRB letters approving them.
- All protocol amendments.
- All IRB updates and notifications including serious adverse events.
- A copy of the IRB membership list.
- A study close out or final report to the IRB.
- All study-related correspondence.
- All drug receipts, records and inventories.
- A telephone log.
- A screening log.

The investigator needs to be meticulous about the upkeep of the loose-leaf book. However, one item that should not be placed in the study binder is your financial contract with the sponsor. This is information that does not need to be available to staff or to the FDA, should it decide to audit your site.

Securing Informed Consent

As described in chapter nine, the investigator must have patients sign an IRB-approved consent form. However, securing informed consent requires more than simply obtaining the patient's signature on the consent form. Good Clinical Practices require that the patient be given an opportunity to discuss what informed consent means. During the discussion, patients should be encouraged to raise any misgivings or concerns they may have about participating in a clinical trial. Both the investigator and the coordinator should be prepared to speak to patients about the benefits and risks associated with participating in the trial. Patients must be told that they will have the right to leave the study at any time. This discussion must be documented in the investigator's progress notes.

The consent form must be signed by the patient and a witness. A family member or the coordinator can serve as a witness. The patient should be given a copy of the form, and the original should be filed with patient's chart. This activity also must be documented in the patient's chart in a note that is signed and dated by the investigator.

Source Documents

In a clinical trial, all information entered on a case report form needs to be supported by source documents. The background source documents for every patient should include:

- Medical history.
- Physical examination results.
- Current medications.
- Medications discontinued in the past 30 days.
- A note that the informed consent form has been signed.
- Telephone logs.
- Appointment books.
- Screening logs.

Every time a patient is seen as part of a clinical trial, a note describing the visit needs to be made part of the source documents. The note can be brief. For example, when a patient is first enrolled, the investigator might write: "patient seen and admitted to protocol #123 sponsored by XXXX. The consent form was discussed and signed. The patient meets the criteria for entrance into the study. Birth control is in the form of a tubal ligation and there are no current meds or allergies. Physical exam was normal except for osteoarthritis of the right knee." The investigator should then sign and date the note.

With every visit, the source-document note should list completed study procedures, treatments received by the patient, and any adverse experiences, illnesses, or problems reported by the patient.

There are other written records that are considered source documents in a clinical trial. The coordinator's appointment book is one. Another is the screening log. The study coordinator must record the name of every patient who has been screened for the study. The "screening" includes a record of patients who have simply been asked whether they would like to participate in the study. For every person screened who decides not to enter the study, an explanatory reason must be given. The patient may not have met the eligibility criteria. Lack of interest is also a perfectly good reason for a screen "failure."

A log that doesn't include many screen failures will immediately raise suspicions. For example, an auditor would immediately question a screen log showing that every person considered for a sore throat study subsequently was found to have a positive strep culture and thus qualified for the study. The experienced auditor would expect that only about 10% of people with sore throats would have a positive strep culture.

Case Report Form

During a study, the coordinator will regularly enter information from the source documents into case report forms. The case report forms are designed by the sponsor to capture trial data that will make it possible to assess the safety and efficacy of the investigational drug. In essence, the final "product" that a site is delivering to the sponsor is a case report form for each patient enrolled in the study.

The case report form is designed by the sponsor. Increasingly, sponsors are using computerized case report forms, as this can speed up the collection and analysis of the data. The computerized data can be submitted to the sponsor on a regular basis throughout the study as well. Regardless of the type of form used, the study coordinator needs to produce case report forms that are as accurate as possible. From the sponsor's point of view, a good site is one that is meticulous about providing clean, complete case report forms. Sites that fail to pay close attention to case report forms cost a sponsor valuable time and money.

The data on the case report forms must be consistent with the source documents. For example, if a case report form states that a patient has a maculopapular rash over his back, this rash must be mentioned in the source documents. This consistency applies to even smaller details. For example, if a patient visit in a source document is listed as having taken place on October 5, 1996, then that same date must be on the case report form. Otherwise, the monitor will question whether the two visits are the same.

Reporting Adverse Events

During the study, the investigator must report all adverse experiences to the sponsor. If an unexpected or serious adverse experience occurs, the investigator must report it immediately to both the sponsor and the governing IRB. As previously stated, all unexpected adverse events must be reported within 24 hours, while serious, but expected, adverse events must be reported within 10 days.

FDA regulations define a serious adverse event as "any experience that suggests a significant hazard, contraindication, side effect or precaution." This includes any experience that is fatal or life threatening, is permanently disabling, requires inpatient hospitalization, or is a congenital anomaly, cancer, or overdose.

This definition needs to be interpreted literally. Furthermore, even if the event is clearly not related to the patient's participation in the clinical trial, it still needs to be reported. For example, if a woman enrolled in an estrogen replacement study is struck by a car while walking across a street, and is hospitalized, the investigator must notify the IRB of this adverse event. The notification is required because the subject required inpatient treatment. (If a patient is not admitted to a hospital, but simply treated in an emergency room, the injury does not qualify as a serious adverse event.)

An "unexpected adverse experience" is defined by the FDA as one that is "not identified in nature, severity, or frequency" in the current investigator brochure; or, if an investigator brochure is not required, that is not identified in nature, severity, or frequency in the risk information described in the general investigational plan or elsewhere in the current application, as amended." An unexpected adverse event must be treated in the same manner as a serious adverse event. The investigator must promptly notify the sponsor and IRB. (If a CRO is being used, the investigator should also inform the CRO of all serious or unexpected adverse events.)

The investigator should always assume responsibility for fulfilling reporting requirements regarding adverse events. An investigator should not rely on the CRO or monitor to report serious or unexpected adverse events to the sponsor and IRB. The investigator should also leave a paper trail documenting that the adverse event has been properly reported. This paper trail includes keeping a log of phone calls to the sponsor and IRB, with each call annotated with time and summary of the discussion.

If there is a question regarding whether a particular event rises to the level of a serious adverse event, it is always better to report it. No investigator will get into trouble by over-reporting. But the failure to report an event that is later deemed serious will be seen as an important omission. An investigator can get into difficulties by failing to report a serious adverse event.

The investigator must also closely document the resolution of any adverse event. The investigator must state the date the adverse experience started, the treatment that was given and the outcome.

Standard Operating Procedures (SOPs)

Today, sites are expected to have a series of SOPs that govern the way they conduct their research. During an audit, the FDA may ask to see these SOPs. The purpose is to standardize the way common procedures are conducted at a site. SOPs should be specific but not so specific as to create issues with their conduct. Things such as consenting patients, drug dispensation, IRB interaction and other typical research processes should be addressed. This SOP book should be accompanied by a log that is signed by every individual involved with the conduct of clinical trials after he or she has read and digested each SOP. The development of SOPs should be an ongoing process where the entire study staff contributes. New SOPs should be discussed at staff meetings and approved by the entire staff. Old SOPs should be reviewed yearly to make sure that they remain relevant.

There are many standard SOP templates available in book or floppy disk format. One such book is *Good Clinical Practice Standard Operating Procedures for Clinical Research* by Josef Kolman and published by John

Wiley & Sons. The Center for Clinical Research Practice has also developed SOP templates for investigative sites. There are others available as well.

Other Study Conduct Tips

Good Medical Practice

Good Clinical Practice describes methods that investigators should follow in order to ensure that the study is conducted in a way that is scientifically valid, and in accordance with all federal regulations and guidelines. At times, however, Good Clinical Practice guidelines can appear to be in conflict with good medical practice. For example, sometimes the appropriate treatment of a particular patient in a study may be precluded by the rigidity of the protocol. Do not try to stretch the limits of the protocol so that the patient can be appropriately treated. The right course is to drop the patient from the study, and treat the patient in accordance with good medical practice. In most instances the investigator will not lose financially because of this decision, and the sponsor will appreciate that the investigator's priorities are in the right order. (It is imperative, of course, that good medical practice take priority over protocol guidelines.)

24-Hour Availability

It is important that a study coordinator or investigator (or a nurse who is knowledgeable about the trial) be accessible at all times. The accessibility can help a site respond promptly to a serious adverse event, should one occur. It also can help a site respond to questions raised by other medical personnel in emergency situations. When an emergency room physician learns that a patient – who may be in the ER for a simple laceration or other ailment unrelated to the study drug – is enrolled in a clinical trial, typically the first thing the physician wants to do is break the medication blind in order to find out what drug the patient is taking. This breaking of the study blind can be prevented only if the ER physician can contact someone who is informed about the clinical trial and can allay any of the physician's concerns.

Many sites have solved this accessibility challenge by having a study coordinator or investigator carry a specific study beeper during the trial. Even if the pager never beeps during the trial, it has still served its purpose. The site has remained accessible throughout the trial.

The Study Blind

Unless it is absolutely necessary, an investigator should never break the study blind. It is not acceptable to do so for reasons of intellectual curiosity or in order to inform the patient which medication he or she received. The study blind should be broken only if not doing so will create a serious or potentially hazardous situation for the patient.

In most instances, a sponsor will unblind the study after it is finished. At that time, the investigator can satisfy his or her own curiosity and also inform the study volunteers whether they received the investigational drug. This type of feedback is important to patients and can help a site recruit them into a subsequent study.

Process versus Outcome

Although I have touched on this previously, it is worth reiterating that a site that gets repeated trials placed with it is one that accommodates the sponsor and the CRO. You must make your site one that responds quickly and accurately to queries and other requests for information. Also, you must accommodate the schedule of the monitors. Make it pleasant for people to deal with your site and make sure that this attitude is prevalent across your organization.

Keeping Staff Interested

As discussed earlier, it is important that you provide incentives to staff that reflect their performance. However, these should not only be monetary in nature. Sometimes the most effective rewards are based on recognition by upper management and that employee's peers. Things as simple as handwritten notes or the purchase of lunch can go a long way to keeping staff motivated. Explore these things because ultimately they are necessary to keep an organization functioning at top performance levels.

 ## Let's Do Lunch

It was the office policy that each time a coordinator completed a trial, the site purchased lunch for the entire staff and brought it into the office. Soon, there was a healthy competition over which coordinator would feed the group most frequently.

Staff Meetings

It is essential that an investigator stays on top of his or her trials. The best way to do this is to have a weekly or bi-weekly staff meeting that gets together all the coordinators, other investigators and other study-related staff. This meeting should be conducted so that the investigator is brought up to speed on all study-related issues including enrollment. An active attempt to identify problems and to solve them should also be a part of this meeting. Staff should be encouraged to voice their opinion and to be as creative as they need to be. This should be an exercise in team building and can be extremely effective if conducted in a creative and open fashion. Also, this type of format can contribute to each individual's self-worth and interest in doing their job. Listen to your staff at these meetings.

Over the past few years, investigators have had to become increasingly self reliant in the conductof clinical trials. It seems that there is less support for sites at both the Sponsor and CRO levels than in the past.

This lack of support manifests itself from the inception and design of the trial, through regulatory submissions, into recruitment and finally through the termination and auditing process.

A Picture is Worth a Thousand Words

If you use an Excel spreadsheet, it is easy to convert numerical information to a graphic form. This is an effective tool to illustrate enrollment numbers and progress to your staff. Chart the projected enrollment against actual enrollment for each current study. This will clearly illustrate to your staff what kind of effort is needed to get the trial back on track.

In a survey conducted by CenterWatch there was a marked decrease in site satisfaction with the interaction of major pharmaceutical sponsors within the USA. While the changes in percentages were not large, the trend was clear and uniformly downward.

Study Specific Responsibilities

Percent of Sites Rating a Typical Sponsor as "Excellent"

	1999	2001
Good Protocol Design	41%	35%
Good CRF Design	36%	34%
Informative Multi-Center Meetings	36%	34%
Efficient Regulatory Process	37%	34%
Efficient Contracting and Budgets	33%	30%
Drug Availability	48%	44%
Patient Recruitment Support	33%	28%
Low Monitor Turnover	37%	38%
Fair Grant Payments	35%	31%
Grant Schedule	35%	28%
Prompt Grant Payments	33%	26%
Efficient Query Handling	30%	27%

Source: CenterWatch 1999, 2001 Surveys of 395 and 405 Investigative Sites, respectively

There is even less support from sponsors outside the top tier and from foreign companies doing research in the United States. This also applies to the CRO industry in general. The reason for the lack of support is that available, experienced, trained personnel are being stretched to a point where functionality is diminished. There are simply not enough trained project managers, monitors and CRAs to support the huge proliferation of new companies and projects.

This trend creates a problem for new sites in that the blind are leading the blind. For example, it would not be unusual for a novice site's CRO contact to be a recent college graduate working on his or her first trial. This individual might also be interfacing with a similarly inexperienced individual at the sponsor. And, in this business, like so many others, there is simply no substitute for experience. There is a great difference between someone who believes they know how to do it and someone who has actually done a trial on multiple occasions before.

This issue makes it more difficult for novice sites to rapidly learn what is needed to become fully functional. Therefore, new sites must depend on other sources of information such as the IRB, other investigators and manuals. The upside is that, in this environment, once a site and its investigator are perceived as competent and knowledgeable, their value is magnified to even a greater extent than in the past. Competent, experienced individuals and sites are worth their weight in gold.

Competition in the Investigator Marketplace

The acceleration of competitive forces in the investigator marketplace is driven partly by narrowing profit margins. More and more physicians look at clinical research as a potential revenue source or simply as something of interest to become involved with.

This trend also is a result of clinical research coming "out of the closet", so to speak. Clinical trials have, in the past few years, gained the notice of the general population. Much of this is a result of the ubiquitous advertising campaigns that are conducted to acquire subjects for trials. On any given ride to the office I will hear at least two or three such ads, some of which are rather creative and professional in nature. These campaigns not only attract patients but also potential investigators.

There are many new and inexperienced individuals at both the sponsors and CROs who have responsibility for site selection. This becomes a major negative for those sites that have performed well and have had long-term relationships with sponsors, as they may be overlooked by newly created project groups. On the other hand, this gives new and inexperienced sites a good chance to become involved in trials, particularly if they are less concerned about the profitability of a given trial.

An additional issue is the globalization of the investigator pool. More trials are being conducted internationally. Sites in France, Holland, the U.K. and other Western European nations have often participated effectively. And, depending on the type of trials, patient requirements and specific regulatory issues, these sites can have some significant advantages or disadvantages in their ability to perform. For example, if a trial involves patients diagnosed with congestive heart failure, a U.K. site may already have a registry of eligible patients, including their classification, simply as a result of the structure of the healthcare system in that country.

Recently, sponsors and CROs have begun to recruit sites in Eastern Europe and have found them extremely cooperative and productive. This also is partially a result of the economic times in those countries. Today both the access to treatment and the fees supplied by clinical trials are at a premium to physicians and patients alike.

A relatively new twist involves the recruitment of investigators in Asia, Central and South America. There is some increasing impetus for sponsors to look to these arenas. First, there are huge populations of untreated and available patients to fill clinical trials. Second, most western nations either already have or are moving toward pricing controls on drug sales. It is, therefore, important for the industry to expand into growing and unregulated areas of the globe for the sale of products. One excellent stratagem is to recruit well known physicians to act as investigators in clinical trials so that in the future they can be called upon as advocates for the product.

Remote Data Entry

The clinical trials industry is slowly transitioning from paper to remote data entry. Currently, however, approximately 95% of all clinical trials are still done with paper, tri-part forms and Federal Express.

There is no doubt that remote electronic data entry (RDE) is a better and more logical approach. The key to the current upswing in interest is that the Web has matured to a point to support worldwide RDE. Before, there were issues in creating interactive networks between sites, CROs, regional CRAs and sponsors that required the establishment of infrastructure involving dedicated lines, hardware and software. Today, all that is required is software because web access is universal and sites can be brought on line utilizing inexpensive wireless technology in areas where phone lines aren't up to the task.

Logic dictates that RDE will be the methodology used to transmit research data in the future. Advantages to the sponsor include instantaneous, real-time access to data at the site allowing the sponsor to make decisions that can save, literally, millions of dollars. These include such critical decisions as "Go – No Go" decisions on new drugs. If a sponsor can get information, even a few weeks early, that allows for the aborting of large-scale trials involving a less promising compound, then the company is in a position to shift funding to a compound that stands a better chance of making it to approval, thereby, making effective use of scarce research funding.

Of course, utilizing software that notifies both the site and the CRA of errors or inconsistencies avoids up to 80% of the queries encountered in a paper system. Again, besides taking months to correct, each query costs a sponsoring company about $115 dollars to correct. Considering that there may be 10,000 of these in a large-scale study, one can readily see that this amounts to real money in very short order.

Then there is the monitoring issue. Utilizing RDE, most of the monitoring including the exchange of information with the coordinator can be accomplished via e-mail, allowing the monitor to function from his or her home office instead of spending time at the site. Actually, the only reason that the monitor would have to visit the site is to check source documentation and to close out the trial.

Larger sponsors have been, however, slow to jump on the RDE bandwagon. This is primarily because it is and always has been, difficult for large organizations to change existing structure and paradigms. Small companies and biotechnology companies are moving much quicker into this area since they are nimbler and less structured. Eventually, though, all will utilize this format because competitive pressures will not be denied, and RDE has the ability to dramatically shorten new compounds' time to market.

Adjusting to RDE has some advantages and disadvantages at the site level. The coordinator generally has instantaneous and continuous access to a monitor so that problems can be dealt with immediately through e-mail interchanges rather than having to revisit them at a less appropriate time. Also, there are fewer monitoring visits to a site. This, therefore, requires less coordinator time and less investigator time. On the other hand, if a site's record keeping is flawed, the opportunities for major disasters to occur are increased.

Another advantage to the site is that RDE should speed up payments because the sponsor and CRO quickly learn when benchmarks, which trigger payments, are reached.

In general, RDE provides many advantages to the site and coordinator. A good system will prevent the coordinator from entering mistakes that will require revisiting and correction later. Also, scheduling of patient visits, sponsor invoicing and other tasks are simplified or removed from her plate. However, RDE will require that each coordinator have access to a computer, preferably right in her study room and that she not be afraid to use it. Some training and support is clearly required, and the investigator needs to insure that his coordinators are trained and up to the task. It goes without saying that Internet access is also required. Welcome to modern times.

Investigator Financial Disclosure

On February 2, 1998, the FDA published final and complete regulations concerning disclosure of any financial interests of clinical investigators, sub investigators and their immediate families, in companies whose products they are actively involved in testing. Essentially, the FDA wants to identify whether there is danger of data being altered, skewed or modified in order to further the finances of "hands on" investigators. Those people who would have the opportunity to alter outcomes.

The FDA is interested in knowing about any "proprietary or equity" interest of the investigator including "ownership interest, stock options, or other financial interests whose value cannot be readily determined" Also the FDA wants to know about any stock in a publicly held company that exceeds

$50,000 dollars as well as any non-study related payments from a sponsor to an investigator that exceed $25,000 dollars.

Generally, an investigator should expect to be asked to disclose any of these arrangements or holdings to the sponsor or CRO, which will then submit form 3454 and/or form 3455 to the FDA for review. To my knowledge, to date, no investigator has been excluded from participation in a clinical trial because of financial conflicts. Of course, the possible of future exclusions does now exist.

There is a copy of the new financial disclosure regulation (sec 54.1) and a published Guidance paper appended to this book if you wish to explore these issues in greater depth.

Site Revenue

Overall, more money is available to investigators than ever before. In the year 2000, the grant market grew at an annual rate of 17%. Pharmaceutical companies, device companies and biotech companies allocated about $3.2 billion for investigator grants. In 1998, the allocation was closer to $2.7 billon. The income for dedicated sites rose dramatically in the year 2000 from approximately $1.14 million per site in 1998 to $1.63 million per site. Also, the average clinical grant increased in value from $52,000 to $56,000.

However, the picture is not quite as rosy as these numbers suggest because studies continue to increase in complexity and, therefore, the cost of conducting these trials rise for the investigator. More procedures are required in each protocol, and patient recruitment may require patients who are harder to recruit. Also, sponsors have more sites to choose from and can be less open to negotiating grants upward.

In this environment, it is possible for an investigator to do better financially than ever before. It is also possible for an investigator to do worse than ever before. There is more money available, which allows for increased profitability if the investigator is both a good manager and discriminatory in his selection of clinical trials. Attention to the details of management and care in negotiating subcontracting elements of the trial become increasingly important. Also, management of your employees' time becomes critical. It's wise to ransfer tasks from highly paid coordinators to less costly office assistants whenever possible as well as to make sure that everyone is using all their time as effectively as possible. It is necessary for the good investigator to become a good manager and businessman. I am not suggesting that you micromanage processes, but it is important to make sure that all your staff keeps their eyes open toward cost savings and the implementation of effective use of their time in everything they do.

Probably, though, the most important factor is the careful analysis of the protocol prior to accepting it. Every aspect, procedure, screening pitfall and other variable must be carefully priced out and calculated. One must be careful to leave margins for error and to make decisions on "worst case" scenarios. If a study is not clearly profitable and there is no other compelling reason to do it (such as interest in an innovative drug, patient needs, or introduction to a new sponsor), then, do not accept it. Wait for the next one.

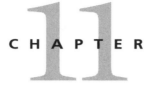

CHAPTER 11

Recruiting Patients

- Courting the Volunteer
- Tapping into Your Own Patient Database
- Speaking to Community Groups
- Newspaper and Radio Ads
- Advertising on the Internet
- Physician Referrals
- Retaining Patients
- Building a Patient Pool

In order to get a new drug approved for market, a pharmaceutical company typically has to conduct trials involving more than 3,000 patients. Recruiting an adequate number of patients to satisfy the FDA is one of the biggest hurdles a pharmaceutical company faces when bringing a new drug to market. Poor patient recruitment is the number one reason that trials fail or are delayed. Between one-half and one-third of all trials fail to meet their enrollment goals.

Sponsor companies may recruit the right sites, but these sites may have over-estimated their potential enrollment. One of the laws of clinical trials states "as soon as you begin a trial for a specific disease entity, you will reduce your encounters with patients having that disease." Some experienced investigators say the best way to cure a disease is to accept a trial for it. But over-estimating enrollment is a serious mistake for the investigator. When a site estimates its ability to participate, the project team counts on it to produce to that level. If the site does not, then the project team looks bad in front of those higher-ups at the company to whom they report. This creates a domino effect of ill will, and I cannot think of a better way to make enemies.

Other potential reasons a trial might fail to recruit are endless. A new drug might have been recently approved that is extremely efficacious for that disease, thereby diminishing patient interest in the trial. The trial might be recruiting during the wrong time of year for that disease process. The requirements to participate in the trial might be so burdensome that no one in their right mind would even consider it. Recruitment might be over the Christmas holidays. There might be multiple competing trials looking for the same patients at the same time. The laboratory process by which cultures are transferred is flawed so no one qualifies for the trial. The patients don't exist.

Because of the many difficulties in enrolling patients, sponsors place a premium on selecting sites that have a good track record of filling their studies. The site that excels at patient recruitment (and also provides good quality data) can be assured that it will get repeat business from sponsors and that its clinical research business will grow. In many ways, success at recruiting patients is what distinguishes the prosperous site from one that muddles along.

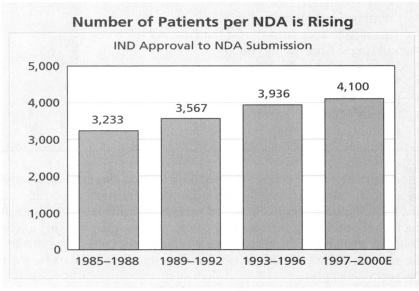

Number of Patients per NDA is Rising

IND Approval to NDA Submission

Source: Boston Consulting Group

In addition to recruiting a specific number of patients, sponsors are increasingly looking for sites that demonstrate they can enroll a diverse range of patients. The FDA is putting pressure on sponsors to test their investigational therapies on the full range of patients who will eventually be using the drug (if it is approved for marketing). As a result, sponsors need to recruit different ethnic groups, men and women, and often people of all ages. The site that fully enrolls its studies, and demonstrates that it can recruit diverse patient groups as well, will quickly win favor with sponsors.

In most instances, in order to fill a study, an investigator will have to use multiple approaches. The site's recruiting practices may vary according to the type of study as well. The recruiting strategies used for a study involving the elderly will be different than the strategies used for recruiting younger patients. The experienced site knows that it is best to develop a recruiting strategy specific to every study it undertakes. The following presents a general strategy for recruiting patients into studies.

Unexpected Stumbling Blocks

I had completed a monilla vaginitis trial a year before, so I was quite certain what my enrollment rate would be. It was also to be enrolled over summer, the best time to find patients with this infection. Last time I had recruited 40 patients in three months, so I was sure that I could put the requested 25 patients in six months into the trial.

I completed the trial with only three patients enrolled. Monistat had come out "over the counter" in the year between these two trials, and no one came to the doctor for treatment of this simple-to-diagnose disorder any more.

Courting the Volunteer

People who volunteer for trials do so for a number of reasons. People with chronic or life-threatening diseases may actively seek out clinical trials as a way to gain early access to promising new drugs. People without health insurance may volunteer for a trial as a way to get free medical care. Some people do it because they like the extra attention they receive. And others agree to participate in a trial because they like the idea that they are doing something to benefit science.

At the same time, people who are considering volunteering for a trial for the first time are likely to have many fears. Are they being used as guinea pigs? Aren't there significant risks? The site that is good at patient recruitment will tap into these various motivations and will help allay these fears. Site personnel will make it clear that the volunteer is valued and address the volunteer's concerns.

This first-class treatment of the study volunteer should begin from the moment of first contact. The initial interview sets the tone for the entire study. The investigative site that takes the time to make the patient feel special and valued during the screening process will find that a remarkably high percentage of people are willing to participate in a clinical trial.

During the initial screening, the investigator or coordinator should sit down with the prospective volunteer and then, in an honest, straightforward manner, discuss exactly what the protocol involves and the potential side effects of the investigational drug. The side-effect profile can be alarming, particularly if the prospective volunteer isn't aware that most drugs already on the market have similar profiles. One way to alleviate these concerns is to let the volunteer read, in the Physicians' Desk Reference, a side-effect profile of drugs they are currently taking or have taken in the past. This will help them put into context the information in the consent form about the potential side effects of the investigational drug.

It is essential to inform prospective volunteers that they will be free to drop out of the trial at any time. The investigator and coordinator may add that they hope that the patient won't drop out for trivial reasons because the sponsor does need to test its drug in patients who remain in the trial to the end. But the clear message should be that patients in a trial may stop at any time and not suffer any consequences. Most prospective volunteers are very relieved to hear this, since it allays their fears. They will be more willing to volunteer once they know they can quit the trial at any time.

At all visits, starting with the initial screening process, the site needs to treat patients with dignity and in a first-class manner. Make sure the patients receive extra consideration and try to keep their waiting to an absolute minimum. If they must wait before a visit, make sure that they are comfortable. Remember: The patient is doing the investigator a service. This is a reversal of the usual paradigm in which the doctor is providing a service to the patient. The investigator and coordinator need to convey a message of gratitude for the volunteer's time and efforts.

As part of this effort, sites should try to show volunteers that they are, in essence, part of a special group. There are a number of ways to do this. A site can acknowledge a volunteer's birthday. Or, if the study involves a chronically ill person who has a caretaker, the site can acknowledge the caretaker's birthday. At the end of a study, a social gathering for all the volunteers can generate remarkable goodwill.

 Guinea Pig Pride

Over the years, more patients than I can count have asked me whether they were being used as guinea pigs. I have always told them that this was true, and at the end of each study they completed, I would give them a t-shirt with a guinea pig prominently displayed across the front. These shirts have become, in a sense, badges of honor. I had the t-shirts made in many different colors, and many of my patients made a point to collect each color.

Tapping into Your Own Patient Database

The best source of patients for most studies is an investigator's own patients. As part of its consideration whether to accept a study, a site should have already reviewed its patient database to identify patients that might be eligible for the study. Once the study is underway, the investigator can recruit from this patient database in several ways.

A site can send a letter to all patients who appear to fit the eligible criteria, informing them of the study and asking them to call if they are interested in learning more. (Remember: any notice sent to patients is considered an advertisement and must be approved first by the IRB. This includes letters, flyers and information presented in any media.)

 That's Why I'm the Doctor

The chief of police was one of my favorite patients. This middle-aged gentleman was always interested in volunteering for trials because he was simply glad to help anyone in any way he could. This particular trial was recruiting patients with osteoarthritis of the hip. Although the chief was complaining of severe pain in his left hip, I felt certain it was not arthritic in nature. In fact, the first thing I did was to remove his huge wallet from his left hip pocket and place it in his right. I immediately cured his pain, but unfortunately, he obviously did not qualify for the trial.

A site can put up a flyer in its general waiting room noting that volunteers are being recruited for a specific study. Unlike the direct mailing, a flyer can help inform all of your patients about the trial. Frequently, patients with ailments unrelated to the study – and thus who would not have received the direct-mail letter – will help spread the word to friends and family members who could be eligible for the study.

The office receptionist needs to be aware of all clinical trials. A patient calling with a complaint relevant to the trial can then be immediately scheduled for a visit. This prompt scheduling is important for two reasons. First, it provides the patient with preferred treatment, and this may encourage the person to volunteer for the trial. Second, it may be required as part of the protocol. For example, a protocol may require that patients be enrolled into the study within 24 hours of the onset of lumbosacral pain. In that case, the receptionist needs to immediately schedule an appointment for anyone calling with a complaint about lower back pain. In a few instances, a site will be able to fully enroll a study from its own patient database. However, it is much more common for an investigator to meet about 50% of his or her patient quota (as called for in the contract), and then to have recruitment stall. The site has fully tapped the potential of its own database and now must recruit from the general population. This presents a separate challenge.

Don't Forget Your Staff

If the atmosphere is right in your office, your staff will be willing to participate in studies. Office staff are ideal candidates for studies that require extended visits. For example, some protocols require blood samples to be taken on an hourly basis for several hours after the administration of the study drug. Since your employees are already at the office, this requirement will not be difficult for them to fulfill. Office staff, of course, are entitled to the same study stipend as other volunteers.

If allowed by the sponsor, it can also be a good idea for an investigator and study coordinator to enroll, at least once, in a study. This way, when a patient asks you (or your study coordinator) if you would ever participate in a trial, you can honestly say that you already have.

Speaking to Community Groups

Reaching out to community groups is an excellent way to recruit patients. Most community groups welcome learning about clinical research. Patient support groups are obvious community groups to target. The study coordinator for a site conducting a diabetes trial can make presentations to local diabetes support groups.

A site should be creative in identifying community groups to address. Patients can be lurking in groups that, at first glance, would have little interest in medical topics. For example, a site conducting a trial involving a vaccine for Lyme disease might make presentations to local hunting, gardening and bird-watching clubs. The study coordinator might also want to send flyers to landscaping firms listed in the yellow pages because they might have employees suffering from Lyme disease.

In addition to being an inexpensive way to recruit patients, speaking to community groups is a good way for an investigator to become more generally known throughout the community as someone who conducts clinical research. This will help the investigator recruit patients for future studies as well.

Newspaper and Radio Ads

In recent years, it has become more common for investigators to use radio and newspaper ads to enhance patient recruitment. The fact that sponsors are willing to pay for this type of expensive advertising exemplifies the importance they are placing on accelerating the clinical development of their new drugs.

STRESS – TENSION – ANXIETY

Halley Medical Center is conducting a study to relieve the symptoms of anxiety using research medications. Your treatment will include a medical evaluation, blood test, EKG and more. You must be over 18.

Call for a confidential evaluation
(943)-7148

In the past, sponsors typically left patient recruitment up to the sites. They would not develop an overall patient-recruitment program to support their sites. This is changing, however. Because of their needs to finish trials more quickly, many sponsors today will organize an overall advertising campaign to support their sites in a large trial. The sponsor may develop general radio and newspaper ads that can be quickly adapted by each site for placement with a local radio station or newspaper.

A few sponsors are now taking their patient-recruitment efforts a step further and hiring advertising agencies to develop television ads to support their sites. Again, the television ad is developed in a flexible manner so it can be easily adapted for local use. When a sponsor employs a patient recruitment firm to do mass marketing, the site must make sure that it interfaces appropriately with the marketing firm. Make sure that you can handle the volume of referral that will be sent to your site. Also, make sure that you don't over-allocate time for these potential referrals, since you don't want to interfere with the normal functioning of your office. Start slowly and adjust your scheduling paradigm frequently when you work with these companies.

If the sponsor does not plan a large-scale recruiting campaign, it usually will still agree to pay for local radio and newspaper ads developed by the site. A site that wants to do local advertising to recruit patients needs to submit this expense as part of its proposed budget. Although a site can often get a sponsor to agree to pay for advertising after the trial is underway, it is best to anticipate this expense and include it in the budget.

Radio, newspaper and television ads will generally produce a steady stream of inquiries from prospective volunteers. It is, however, important to judiciously place ads. A radio ad for an Alzheimer's study that runs on a punk rock station isn't likely to produce any volunteers. But a radio ad for an Alzheimer's study that runs in the middle of a talk show addressing elderly health issues is likely to be very productive. In a similar vein, an ad in a local neighborhood newspaper might be much more cost-effective than placing an ad in a big metropolitan paper. As part of its advertising efforts, a site needs to seek advice on the best place and time for its ads to run.

The downside to advertising in general media outlets is that often most of the people who respond don't qualify for the study. A well-placed radio

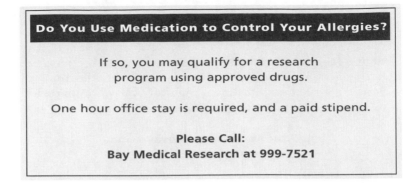

or television spot may generate 100 calls to be screened, but only one or two patients eligible for the study. If this happens, the site incurs significant expense answering the calls and bringing prospective volunteers in for screening visits. In order to be cost-effective, radio, newspaper and television ads need to communicate, as much as possible, the specific therapeutic category involved, since this will help reduce the number of inappropriate calls.

In order to make the best use of advertising dollars, a site should track all patient inquiries and determine how the responders heard about the trial. The tracking will help a site evaluate the effectiveness of advertising in different mediums and how effective advertising can be for different types of studies. Not all studies lend themselves to recruiting different patients through advertisements. The tracking will also enable a site to become better at placing ads in a cost-effective manner.

Advertising on the Internet

A relatively new avenue for reaching patients is the Internet. The Internet has become a popular resource for people with chronic illnesses searching for medical information. Patient-support groups on America Online and throughout the Internet community regularly share information about opportunities to participate in clinical trials.

There are several ways a site can use the Internet to recruit patients. The site can set up its own web page and put up information about all of its trials. The problem with a site doing it on its own is that the web is a very noisy place today, and patients will have a difficult time finding your web site.

A site can also put its trials on other web sites that carry information about clinical research. The CenterWatch Trials Listing Service on the Internet (www.centerwatch.com) carries information about more than 7,000 research trials and is visited by more than 150,000 patients monthly. Patients can use the CenterWatch site to search for trials by both geographic region and therapeutic category. This search mechanism enables patients to identify investigators in their communities who are doing research that may be of interest to them.

Because a site can list the inclusion-exclusion criteria as part of its description of the trial, a posting on the Internet should not generate a large number of inquiries from patients who are not eligible for the study. Advertising on the Internet is also much less expensive than radio, newspaper or television advertising. However, it is not likely to generate the same volume of inquiries as radio, newspaper or television ads. Posting information about your research on the Internet should be seen as a way to supplement your regular patient-recruitment efforts.

Physician Referrals

At times, investigators will appeal to other physicians in their communities for patients.If the investigational drug is particularly innovative, and is for a chronic condition that cannot be effectively treated with drugs already on the market, this appeal may generate a few patients. However, in today's competitive healthcare environment, physicians are usually reluctant to refer patients to an investigator conducting clinical trials. They don't want to lose the income or their patients.

One way to get around this is to negotiate an agreement with another area physician to serve as a sub-investigator on your trial. This can help you deliver more patients. However, this can present practical problems. In some instances, it will be difficult to split the study drug because of randomization issues. The principal investigator who utilizes a sub-investigator must also pay careful attention to regulatory issues and source documentation. Most sponsors also prefer that an investigator not utilize sub-investigators who practice at different sites.

Retaining Patients

Many sites breathe a sigh of relief when they have enrolled patients into a study. The hard part of patient-recruitment seems to have been accomplished. Unfortunately, enrolling patients into a study is only half the battle. The other challenge is retaining them throughout the study.

There are a number of ways that a site can encourage patients to remain in a study until the end. Any and all efforts to treat patients as special will go a long way to achieving this goal. Birthday cards, as mentioned earlier, can work wonders. Here are some other practical tips:

- The stipend for the study should cover a patient's out-of-pocket expenses and perhaps provide a small payment for the patient's time. A typical stipend may pay for $15 to $25 per office visit. Although this isn't much, for some people it still can provide an extra financial incentive for enrolling in a trial and completing all study visits.

■ The site should ensure that volunteers' transportation needs are met. This may involve paying for taxis or even operating a van to transport elderly patients to and from the office. Some volunteers may not own cars and must rely on public transportation; a site should be aware of this and take steps to provide the necessary transportation or cover the associated expense.

■ If a protocol requires the enrollment of women volunteers, a site may need to provide some type of on-site day care. This is particularly true if the protocol will require the patient to stay in the office for an extended period. Even if the visits are short, a site needs to provide appropriate reading or play materials in the waiting room for the children.

■ Patients in a clinical trial are usually required to come to the office for a checkup at fairly precise intervals. It is important that patients not miss a visit. A site that reminds volunteers with a telephone call a day ahead of scheduled visits can greatly increase patient compliance. Periodic telephone calls also can be used to encourage patients to take the study drug at scheduled times.

All of these patient-retention tips flow from a single concept, one that bears repeating: the patient is doing you a favor. As long as that is your guiding premise, you will be motivated to treat the volunteers in a way that makes them feel valued and encourages them to remain in the study to the end.

Carrying Patients

As an investigator, it was my practice to carry a group of patients between studies, particularly patients who had proven to be dedicated and reliable study volunteers. This worked best for hypertensive studies. We had patients who went from study to study over the course of several years. (There would have to be an appropriate washout period between studies, of course. In general, patients must have at least 30 days between studies.)

Generally, we would supply these patients with free medications and treatments between studies. On average, at any given time, we would carry between 50 and 100 hypertensive patients.

These patients became quite sophisticated about hypertension, and often would be quite analytical about the studies. Some patients, for example, would only participate in studies involving ACE inhibitors.

Building a Patient Pool

Volunteers who have successfully completed a trial are often very receptive to participating in other trials as well. Their fears and concerns about clinical research have been allayed by their first experience, and they may have enjoyed the attention they received as study volunteers. A site should be constantly building a database of "trial volunteers" that can be tapped for all future studies.

The information on every volunteer in this database should include the type of trial the patient participated in, whether the patient completed the trial, and any other pathologies or conditions the patient may have. For example, a person with asthma may have participated in a diabetes trial. A trial database should list that person under both asthma and diabetes. Thus, if the site subsequently secures a grant for an asthma study, it can immediately inquire whether the person would be interested in volunteering. The study may be different, but the person is already familiar with the general process of clinical research.

Again, in the long run, any site's success is dependent upon the successful recruitment and retention of patients. The best sites are ones that have developed creative and innovative approaches to this patient-recruitment challenge.

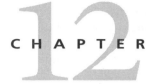

CHAPTER

Evaluating Your Performance

- Short Start-Up Times
- Evaluable Patients
- Quality Data
- Other Questions
- Your Evaluation

A fter a study is completed, many sponsors will assess the performance of the sites. Sites that have performed well will get future grants; those that performed below the norm probably will not.

A site should fill out its own after-study report card as well. This self-evaluation will enable a site to pinpoint areas in which it needs to improve and will also provide it with performance data that can be used – if a site regularly performs well – for marketing purposes.

In general, sponsors are evaluating site performance in three categories. A site's self-assessment should focus on these three areas.

Short Start-Up Times

In recent years, pharmaceutical companies have placed a great emphasis on shortening the time it takes to develop a new drug. Even cutting off a month of development time can bring a pharmaceutical company millions of dollars in additional revenues. As a result, pharmaceutical companies today want to select sites that can start studies very quickly.

In general, physicians at academic medical centers take much longer to start studies than do physicians in community settings. One industry survey, published in 1995, found that academic physicians typically took two to five months to complete budget and contract negotiations and obtain IRB approval to do the study. In contrast, community physicians often completed this process in one to four weeks.

This time disparity is one reason pharmaceutical companies began placing more trials with community physicians. In response, academic medical centers have been shortening their study start-up times. The market message is clear: In today's competitive environment, a site needs to have the administrative machinery in place to start a research trial in a few weeks.

A site's self-evaluation should assess how long it took to review and approve the contract, prepare a budget, and obtain IRB approval. An experienced site that isn't affiliated with an academic center should try to complete these tasks within seven to 10 days. Although it may be impossible for an investigator at an academic medical center to fulfill these chores within 10 days, the investigator should still seek to complete them within a month. An academic investigator who takes much longer than this will be viewed as working at an institution that has not found a way to nurture industry-sponsored clinical research.

Evaluable Patients

If clinical research were an easy enterprise, sites would routinely meet their patient quotas. They would recruit the number of patients called for in the contract and would finish the study on time.

Unfortunately, that scenario is the exception rather than the rule. Studies are regularly delayed or extended because sites encounter difficulties in meeting their full patient quotas. At industry conferences, speakers representing pharmaceutical companies regularly tell of studies where the majority of sites failed miserably in meeting their patient quotas.

Much of this poor performance may not be the site's fault. A protocol's inclusion-exclusion criteria may be so strict that sites find it very difficult to identify patients who fit the criteria. But remember: a site reviews protocol before signing a contract. It can anticipate the difficulties of recruiting and retaining patients, and, in order to not oversell itself, contract to test the investigational drug in a relatively small number of patients. If it reaches this smaller target goal, the site will still be evaluated by the sponsor as having delivered 100% of the number of patients called for in the contract.

It is this patient-quota percentage – rather than absolute numbers – that should be the metric a site uses for its own self-assessment. Did it meet – or even exceed – its patient quota? A site that develops a track record of regularly meeting its patient quota (or at least coming close), will be seen as a superior site.

Also, as a site examines its performance in this area, it should focus on evaluable patients, rather than on patients enrolled. A patient who enrolls in a trial and then drops out for a non-medical reason may not provide the sponsor with any data it can use. The dropout patient is simply an added expense. An evaluable patient is one who has completed the study or who had to be taken off the investigational drug for a medical reason. In bottom-line terms, the product a site delivers to a sponsor is data for evaluable patients – data that can support a new drug application to the FDA. Thus, for its own internal report card, a site should look at the number of evaluable patients it delivered to the sponsor to assess whether it met its patient quota.

Quality Data

Throughout a study, a monitor will visit the sites to review their case report forms. During these visits, the monitor will flag any omissions or errors in the case report forms, a process that helps keep the case report forms in good order as the trial progresses. Even so, after the study has ended, and all the participating sites have submitted their final case report forms, the sponsor may still take months in "cleaning" the data. During this process, the sponsor will raise new questions that the sites must answer.

Naturally, sponsors are now using this data-cleaning process to develop a rough metric for evaluating the quality of data submitted by a site. On a particular study, a sponsor may determine how many questions it raised for each case report form submitted by a site, and calculate an average number of queries per case report form for all sites in the study. Sites that beat this average (e.g., had a low number of queries per case report form) are seen as having provided high-quality data.

The limitation with this measure is that not all queries are equal. Was the omission or error that triggered the query significant? Or was it a simple typographical error? Was the query really the fault of the site? Or did the site get poor instructions on filling out the case report form?

Although queries-per-case-report-form is only a rough measure of quality, it is still the best measure available today. Therefore, a site should track its own performance in this regard. On a particular study, what was its number of queries per case report form? If possible, the site should ask the sponsor for the average number of queries per case report form for all sites in the study. Did your site do better than the average? Or worse?

Other Questions

In addition to gathering the performance data detailed above, a site's post-study assessment might include two other items.

It can be a good idea to ask the lead monitor on the study to provide a review of your site's performance. Was your site easy to work with? During visits to your site, did the monitor find that his or her work space was acceptable? Was your site responsive to the monitor's questions? Asking a monitor to fill out a survey will provide your site with additional feedback on your performance and will also be a signal that you value the monitor's opinion. Most monitors will appreciate this interest.

Your checklist should include reviewing whether you have inquired about future grant opportunities. Did you ask the monitor about any upcoming trials? Did you ask the project manager about upcoming trials? A study typically lasts from several months to more than a year. This has given a site ample time and opportunity to market itself to the sponsor and CRO. At the end of the study, the monitor and project manager should know more about the full extent of your capabilities and your interest in clinical research.

Your Evaluation

It is also important for a site to evaluate its own progress regarding both financial and productivity aspect from its own viewpoint. This might be an exercise that is best accomplished on a yearly basis.

First, your best evidence that you are building a research business is the growth of the enterprise. Are you getting new trials, and are you completing them? Are you getting trials from new companies, and are you getting repeat business? Obviously, you will have a feel for how you are doing, but it is important to actually apply metrics to it. Create a couple of spreadsheets and convert them to graphics. Develop a feel for your past growth so that you can anticipate future growth. Then staff and build accordingly.

It is likely, if your endeavor is proceeding well, that you have obtained at least four trials your first year. A successful site should be able to double this the next year and possibly double it again in year three. Of course, there are mitigating factors, but, overall, the trend should be upward.

Measure your success in filling each trial. Measure this against the other sites in the trial as well as against what you have promised the sponsor. This information is not only of critical importance to you but can be translated into advertising ammunition that can be sent to sponsors and CROs in marketing letters.

Also, do not neglect the fiscal component of the business. Track your revenue and derive a net figure. Track your costs, and look at overall profit trends. As you earn enough to cover fixed costs, your profit margin should begin to grow. If not, you need to know why. Perhaps you are overstaffing, or perhaps you are paying too much for advertising. Maybe an SMO is involved and taking too large a slice of the profits. Track, break down and measure this. Use your computer and the spreadsheet programs to slice and dice this information. If your site is not becoming increasingly profitable as you do more trials, there is clearly something broken. In reality, your new company should be in the black sometime in year two.

Look at the finances of each trial separately. Figure out your costs and profit on each trial and then apply this information when bidding for future work of a similar nature. There may actually be reasons to take very little or no profit on particular trials. For example, if you are very interested in working with a new compound, or if you want to work with a new company, it is all right to take a loss on a trial if it ultimately will bring in more profitable work in the future. What isn't all right is to lose money unintentionally. This is something you can't make up with volume.

Finally, apply the metrics to your advertising. Figure out where you get the best bang for your buck. Do the same with employee productivity. Ask your accountant for other indices that need to be measured, but, to ultimately be successful, you need to develop and apply business principles and measurements to your clinical trials business.

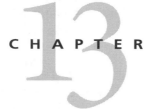

CHAPTER

Anticipating An Audit

A ny investigator who conducts clinical trials on a regular basis will
eventually be audited by the sponsoring company, the CRO and
probably, the FDA.

Company or CRO audits are fairly common. Usually companies audit
trials that are considered pivotal. These trials are very important for the support of the NDA, and these are trials that it is likely that the FDA will audit.

It is wise to consider a sponsor audit as a positive event. First, when
deficiencies are discovered in the course of these audits, the site has ample
opportunity to correct them prior to an FDA audit. Second, this audit should
be viewed as a great learning tool for the site. Here you have the chance to see
how good you are. And, if there are problems uncovered, the site has a chance
to correct them in this trial and then to apply that knowledge to future trials. Company audits, if properly utilized, are a site's best tool for self-improvement. Finally, if your audit is good, it is likely that everyone at the
sponsoring company and CRO will know about it. This can prove to be a
most effective marketing tool.

FDA audits are a little different. The most common type of audit is a routine surveillance inspection. The second is a for-cause audit. Most sites never
experience a for-cause audit. A for-cause audit suggests that questions may
have been raised about the site's integrity. One thing that triggers a surveillance audit is if the data from your site differs slightly from the data collected from every other site. A second reason might be that you are the highest
enroller in a particular trial. A site is particularly likely to be audited in this
manner if it has enrolled a large number of patients in a pivotal study.

The FDA uses the routine surveillance inspections to verify that the data submitted by a pharmaceutical company to support an NDA is reliable data. The FDA also uses these inspections to ensure that the study was conducted in a manner that did not jeopardize the study subjects or compromise their rights.

To schedule an audit, an FDA inspector will call the site and ask to schedule a time he or she can visit. Normally, the inspector will want to visit within two weeks. As soon as a site receives the initial call, it should notify the pharmaceutical company that sponsored the study. The study coordinator will need to retrieve the study documents from storage as well. (Often, the audit will be for a study that was completed one or two years ago. As discussed earlier in this book, a site needs to store records for completed studies in a sealed banker's box.)

Upon arrival at the site, the FDA inspector must show credentials or a badge. The inspector should be provided with a quiet place to work. The inspector's questions should be answered specifically, but not elaborated upon. The inspector should not be allowed to take original documents from the site, nor should the inspector be given information concerning financial contracts. If a site has a question about whether a particular request by the FDA inspector is appropriate, it should call the sponsor. The sponsor's regulatory staff can provide assistance.

The audit may last from a few hours to as long as a week. At the conclusion, the inspector will conduct an exit interview. The auditor will review any inconsistencies or questions with the investigator and give the investigator form FDA-483. This form will list any deficiencies that were found.

A few weeks later, the FDA will send a letter to the site reviewing its findings. In the letter the FDA will make one of three determinations. The first, and most favorable, is that it did not discover any deficiencies. This type of finding occurs infrequently and of course requires no follow up from the site. Letters like this are of tremendous value in future marketing campaigns for your site. Copy it and distribute it to future potential sponsors.

The second determination, which is the most common, is that some minor deviations were found. Although the site will need to remedy the deficiencies in future studies, it doesn't need to make any further response to the FDA. This second finding is basically a "we all make mistakes" letter.

The third possible determination, which can spell serious trouble for an investigator, is called a "notice of adverse findings." This notice is sent after serious deficiencies have been discovered during an audit. The investigator must respond in writing. A notice of adverse findings may force the sponsor to disregard the site's trial data in its analysis of study results. It also may lead to a for-cause audit.

A for-cause audit does not necessarily mean that a site is in trouble. A site that enrolls an inordinately high number of patients in a pivotal trial may find itself the subject of a for-cause audit. However, a for-cause audit always needs to be treated in a serious fashion. A for-cause audit may be triggered because data generated at your site is inconsistent with the data from all the other sites in a study, or inconsistent with laboratory data, or doesn't appear to be believable. A for-cause audit may also be caused by a suggestion of fraud at your site from the sponsor or monitor.

A for-cause audit is conducted in much the same manner as a surveillance inspection, except that the audit is much more in-depth. Usually, the FDA will send two auditors to your site, including a scientist from FDA's headquarters. If the auditors uncover fraudulent or deceptive practices, the investigator will face serious sanctions. The investigator may be blacklisted, which precludes further participation in clinical research. The FDA may also criminally prosecute investigators for fraudulent practices.

The prospect of any audit can make an investigator uncomfortable. However, it is important to realize that an investigator will not get into trouble for honest mistakes. No one expects a site to turn in absolutely perfect work. The number of investigators who stray from this honest path and are blacklisted for fraud, is small.

When the FDA comes to your site for an audit, there are appropriate ways to deal with the auditor. Sponsoring companies normally advise that the auditor be made comfortable but not dealt with in an overly friendly manner. One auditor told me that his usual technique in doing an audit involved making friends with a member of the staff who was not necessarily directly involved in the conduct of research. This connection was then exploited to hunt for any damaging information. So, be polite, but do not allow the auditor free run of the office or free interchange with your staff.

It is important that you as the investigator be present for the full period that an FDA inspector is at your site. This is for two reasons. First, the inspector will only perceive that the trial is important to you if you make the effort to be there. Second, you want to be the one either to give answers to the inspector or to determine which of your staff will.

The most common observations that result from an audit include the following:

1. Source documents differ from the information contained in the case report form.
2. Protocol-required procedures were not completed.
3. Visit intervals as specified on the protocol were violated.
4. Concomitant medications were not reported.
5. All IRB correspondence was not found.
6. Drug inventory records were incorrect.
7. Consents were not properly signed, dated and witnessed.
8. All Investigational New Drug safety reports were not found.
9. Inclusion and exclusion criteria were not followed.
10. All investigator CVs were not on file.

It is clear that most of these issues are totally avoidable if the proper attention is applied to the trial process.

Questions about your conduct of a trial may be forwarded to the FDA by the sponsor, the CRO, a patient or the IRB. However, the individual most likely to notify the FDA is a current or former employee. Frequently, it is a coordinator, lab tech or an office manager who has been forced to participate in a fraudulent process against his or her conscience.

This is exactly what happened to an investigator in California recently. A physician was apparently substituting urine samples so that patients who did not qualify were allowed into the trial. This was in addition to actually fabricating patients completely. That investigator is currently in federal prison looking for protocols to conduct in that venue.

One quarter of all complaints filed with the FDA is related to protocol violations. An additional quarter is complaints suggesting that data falsification has occurred. The next largest category is complaints involving the consent form and consenting process, and the fourth major category is complaints involving failure to report adverse events.

Over the past few years the FDA has significantly increased its response to complaints by increasing the numbers of inspections. In 1998, about 40 inspections occurred due to complaints. In 2000, that number increased by 50% to 60 inspections.

Any hint of impropriety or fraud in the conduct of a trial is something that immediately closes the door on any future relationship with a sponsor or CRO. And, it is not uncommon for discussions about any potential fraudulent behavior to occur at the highest level in a research organization.

It is important for investigators to understand how intimately upper management is involved in each clinical trial, particularly if it is pivotal in nature. Enrollment figures and site performance are reviewed at each steering committee meeting for these trials. The sponsor company's senior management can be present. You, as an investigator, are recognized from the highest level in a company all the way down to the CRA. There is no anonymity. This can work in your favor if you perform well. On the other hand, it is absolutely deadly if there is any hint of fraudulent behavior. Fraud, even at one site, can derail an entire NDA. Depending on the statistical significance of a particular site, the entire trial may need to be rerun in addition to any other trials that that particular investigator had participated in. Fraud in an investigation is one of the most devastating events that a pharmaceutical company can encounter.

Closing Remarks

Clinical research can be an exciting and stimulating addition to a medical practice. Benefits to physician, staff and patients can occur in numerous ways as a result of involvement. It also is one of the few bastions of capitalism that still exists in medicine today. Clinical research can be an extraordinarily lucrative pursuit for the physician if done properly. The trick is to do it right both from a medical perspective and a business one. I hope this book has given you some of the tools you need to make this work.

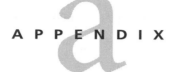

APPENDIX

Industry Resources

Associations

- **Association of Clinical Research Professionals (ACRP)**
  1012 14th Street NW, Suite 807
  Washington, DC 20005
  (202) 737-8100
  www.acrp.net

- **Drug Information Association (DIA)**
  501 Office Center Drive, Suite 450
  Fort Washington, PA 19034
  (215) 628-2288
  www.diahome.org

- **Pharmaceutical Research and Manufacturers of America (PhRMA)**
  1100 Fifteenth Street NW
  Washington DC 20005
  (202) 835-3400
  www.phrma.org

Conference Organizers

- **Barnett International**
  Rose Tree Corporate Center
  1400 North Providence Road, Suite 2000
  Media, PA 19063-2043
  (800) 856-2556
  www.barnettinternational.com

- **Center for Business Intelligence (CBI)**
  500 West Cummings Park, Suite 5100
  Woburn, MA 01801
  (781) 939-2400
  www.cbinet.com

- **Institute for International Research (IIR)**
  708 3rd Avenue, 4th Floor
  New York, NY 10017
  (212) 661-3500
  www.iir.org

- **International Quality and Productivity Center**
  150 Clove Road
  PO Box 401
  Little Falls, NJ 07424-0401
  (800) 882-8684
  www.iqpc.com

- **SRI International**
  333 Ravenswood Avenue
  Menlo Park, CA 94025
  (800) 982-8655
  www.sri.com

Publishers

- **Advanstar Communications**
  859 Willamette Street
  Eugene, OR 97401
  (541) 343-1200
  www.advanstar.com
  Publications include *Applied Clinical Trials* and *Pharmaceutical Executive.*

- **CenterWatch**
  22 Thomson Place
  Boston, MA 02210
  (617) 856-5900
  www.centerwatch.com
  Publications include newsletters such as *CenterWatch Monthly, CW Weekly, CenterWatch Europe, JobWatch,* and *New Medical Therapies,* as well as a wide range of directories and manuals.

- **CTB International Publishing, Inc.**
  PO Box 218
  Maplewood, NJ 07040
  (973) 379-7749
  www.ctbintl.com
  Publications include *Clinical Trials Monitor, Biotechnology News, Diagnostics Intelligence, Clinical Investigator News* and *Emerging Pharmaceuticals*

- **Engel Publishing Partners**
  820 Bear Tavern Road
  West Trenton, NJ 08628
  (609) 530-0044
  Publications include MedAd News and R&D Directions.

- **F-D-C Reports, Inc.**
  5550 Friendship Boulevard, Suite One
  Chevy Chase, MD 20815-7278
  (800) 332-2181
  www.fdcreports.com
  Publications include *The Pink Sheet* and *The Tan Sheet.*

- **PJB Publications Ltd.**
  Pharma Books (U.S. Office)
  1775 Broadway, Suite 511
  New York, NY 10019
  (212) 262-8230
  www.pjbpubs.com
  Publications include *Scrip Reports, Scrip Magazine, Scrip Yearbook* and *Pharmaprojects.*

- **Research Investigator's Source, Inc. (RIS)**
  715 Florida Avenue South, Suite 105
  Minneapolis, MN 55426
  (763) 591-7790
  www.clinicalinvestigators.com
  Publications include an industry directory.

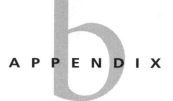

APPENDIX

Top Sponsors

- **American Home Products**
  5 Giralda Farms
  Madison, NJ 07940
  (973) 660-5000
  www.ahp.com
  Research & Development Division:
  Wyeth-Ayerst

- **AstraZeneca**
  1800 Concord Pike
  Wilmington, DE 19850
  (302) 886-3000
  www.astrazeneca.com

- **Bristol-Myers Squibb**
  345 Park Avenue
  New York, NY 10154-0037
  (212) 546-4000
  www.bms.com

- **Eli Lilly**
  Lilly Corporate Center
  Indianapolis, IN 46285
  (317) 276-4000
  www.lilly.com

- **GlaxoSmithKline**
  5 Moore Drive
  Research Triangle Park, NC 27709
  or
  One Franklin Plaza
  Philadelphia, PA 19102
  (888) 825-5249
  www.gsk.com

- **Hoechst Marion Roussel**
  10236 Marion Park Drive
  Kansas City, MO 64137-1405
  (816) 966-4000
  www.hoechst.com

- **Johnson & Johnson**
  One Johnson & Johnson Plaza
  New Brunswick, NJ 08933
  (732) 524-0400
  www.jnj.com
  Research & Development Divisions:
  Ortho-McNeil
  Robert W. Johnson Pharmaceutical Research Institute
  Janssen Pharmaceutica

- **Merck**
  One Merck Drive
  Whitehouse Station, NJ 08889-0100
  (908) 423-1000
  www.merck.com

- **Novartis**
  556 Morris Avenue
  Summit, NJ 07901
  (973) 783-8300
  www.novartis.com

- **Pfizer**
  235 East 42nd Street
  New York, NY 10017-5755
  (212) 573-2323
  www.pfizer.com

Top Contract Research Organizations (CROS)

- **aai Pharma** (includes the former MTRA)
  2320 Scientific Park Drive
  Wilmington, NC 28405
  (800) 575-4AAI
  www.aaiintl.com

- **Covance**
  210 Carnegie Center
  Princeton, NJ 08540
  (888) COVANCE
  www.covance.com

- **Inveresk Research** (includes the former ClinTrials)
  11000 Weston Parkway, Suite 100
  Cary, NC 27513
  (800) 988-9845
  www.inveresk.com

- **Kendle International Inc.**
  1200 Carew Tower
  Cincinnati, OH 45202
  (800) 733-1572
  www.kendle.com

- **MDS Pharma** (includes the former Phoenix International)
  2350 Cohen Street
  Saint-Laurent, Quebec H4R 2N6 Canada
  (514) 333-0033
  www.mdsps.com

- **Omnicare Clinical Research**
  630 Allendale Road
  King of Prussia, PA 19406
  (800) 290-5766
  www.omnicare.com

- **PPD**
  3151 South 17th Street
  Wilmington, NC 28412
  (910) 251-0081
  www.ppdi.com

- **PRA International, Inc.**
  8300 Greensboro Drive, Suite 400
  McLean, VA 22102
  (703) 748-0760
  www.praintl.com

- **Parexel International**
  195 West Street
  Waltham, MA 02451
  (781) 487-9900
  www.parexel.com

- **Premier Research Worldwide**
  30 South 17th Street
  Philadelphia, PA 19103
  (215) 282-5500
  www.scp.com

- **Quintiles Transnational**
  PO Box 13979
  Research Triangle Park, NC 27709-3979
  (919) 998-2000
  www.quintiles.com

Performance Measures

Speed

- Number of patients by indication
- Average number of patients enrolled per week
- Average contract and/or protocol review and approval times
- Number of studies coordinator has conducted

Quality

- CRF legibility
- Average number of studies conducting currently
- Ease with which patient records accessed

Cost

- Procedural and overhead cost comparables
- Budget preparation and negotiation efficiency

APPENDIX

World Medical Association Declaration of Helsinki

Ethical Principles for Medical Research Involving Human Subjects

A. Introduction

1. The World Medical Association has developed the Declaration of Helsinki as a statement of ethical principles to provide guidance to physicians and other participants in medical research involving human subjects. Medical research involving human subjects includes research on identifiable human material or identifiable data.

2. It is the duty of the physician to promote and safeguard the health of the people. The physician's knowledge and conscience are dedicated to the fulfillment of this duty.

3. The Declaration of Geneva of the World Medical Association binds the physician with the words, "The health of my patient will be my first consideration," and the International Code of Medical Ethics declares that, "A physician shall act only in the patient's interest when providing medical care which might have the effect of weakening the physical and mental condition of the patient."

4. Medical progress is based on research which ultimately must rest in part on experimentation involving human subjects.

5. In medical research on human subjects, considerations related to the well-being of the human subject should take precedence over the interests of science and society.

6. The primary purpose of medical research involving human subjects is to improve prophylactic, diagnostic and therapeutic procedures and the understanding of the aetiology and pathogenesis of disease. Even the best proven prophylactic, diagnostic, and therapeutic methods must continuously be challenged through research for their effectiveness, efficiency, accessibility and quality.

7. In current medical practice and in medical research, most prophylactic, diagnostic and therapeutic procedures involve risks and burdens.

8. Medical research is subject to ethical standards that promote respect for all human beings and protect their health and rights. Some research populations are vulnerable and need special protection. The particular needs of the economically and medically disadvantaged must be recognized. Special attention is also required for those who cannot give or refuse consent for themselves, for those who may be subject to giving consent under duress, for those who will not benefit personally from the research and for those for whom the research is combined with care.

9. Research Investigators should be aware of the ethical, legal and regulatory requirements for research on human subjects in their own countries as well as applicable international requirements. No national ethical, legal or regulatory requirement should be allowed to reduce or eliminate any of the protections for human subjects set forth in this Declaration.

B. Basic Principles for All Medical Research

10. It is the duty of the physician in medical research to protect the life, health, privacy, and dignity of the human subject.

11. Medical research involving human subjects must conform to generally accepted scientific principles, be based on a thorough knowledge of the scientific literature, other relevant sources of information, and on adequate laboratory and, where appropriate, animal experimentation.

12. Appropriate caution must be exercised in the conduct of research which may affect the environment, and the welfare of animals used for research must be respected.

13. The design and performance of each experimental procedure involving human subjects should be clearly formulated in an experimental protocol. This protocol should be submitted for consideration, comment, guidance, and where appropriate, approval to a specially appointed ethical review committee, which must be independent of the investigator, the sponsor or any other kind of undue influence. This independent committee should be in conformity with the laws and regulations of the country in which the research experiment is performed. The committee has the right to monitor ongoing trials. The researcher has the obligation to provide monitoring information to the committee, especially any serious adverse events. The researcher should also submit to the committee, for review, information regarding funding, sponsors, institutional affiliations, other potential conflicts of interest and incentives for subjects.

14. The research protocol should always contain a statement of the ethical considerations involved and should indicate that there is compliance with the principles enunciated in this Declaration.

15. Medical research involving human subjects should be conducted only by scientifically qualified persons and under the supervision of a clinically competent medical person. The responsibility for the human subject must always rest with a medically qualified person and never rest on the subject of the research, even though the subject has given consent.

16. Every medical research project involving human subjects should be preceded by careful assessment of predictable risks and burdens in comparison with foreseeable benefits to the subject or to others. This does not preclude the participation of healthy volunteers in medical research. The design of all studies should be publicly available.

17. Physicians should abstain from engaging in research projects involving human subjects unless they are confident that the risks involved have been adequately assessed and can be satisfactorily managed. Physicians should cease any investigation if the risks are found to outweigh the potential benefits or if there is conclusive proof of positive and beneficial results.

18. Medical research involving human subjects should only be conducted if the importance of the objective outweighs the inherent risks and burdens to the subject. This is especially important when the human subjects are healthy volunteers.

19. Medical research is only justified if there is a reasonable likelihood that the populations in which the research is carried out stand to benefit from the results of the research.

20. The subjects must be volunteers and informed participants in the research project.

21. The right of research subjects to safeguard their integrity must always be respected. Every precaution should be taken to respect the privacy of the subject, the confidentiality of the patient's information and to minimize the impact of the study on the subject's physical and mental integrity and on the personality of the subject.

22. In any research on human beings, each potential subject must be adequately informed of the aims, methods, sources of funding, any possible conflicts of interest, institutional affiliations of the researcher, the anticipated benefits and potential risks of the study and the discomfort it may entail. The subject should be informed of the right to abstain from participation in the study or to withdraw consent to participate at any time without reprisal. After ensuring that the subject has understood the information, the physician should then obtain the subject's freely-given informed consent, preferably in writing. If the consent cannot be obtained in writing, the non-written consent must be formally documented and witnessed.

23. When obtaining informed consent for the research project the physician should be particularly cautious if the subject is in a dependent relation-

ship with the physician or may consent under duress. In that case the informed consent should be obtained by a well-informed physician who is not engaged in the investigation and who is completely independent of this relationship.

24. For a research subject who is legally incompetent, physically or mentally incapable of giving consent or is a legally incompetent minor, the investigator must obtain informed consent from the legally authorized representative in accordance with applicable law. These groups should not be included in research unless the research is necessary to promote the health of the population represented and this research cannot instead be performed on legally competent persons.

25. When a subject deemed legally incompetent, such as a minor child, is able to give assent to decisions about participation in research, the investigator must obtain that assent in addition to the consent of the legally authorized representative.

26. Research on individuals from whom it is not possible to obtain consent, including proxy or advance consent, should be done only if the physical/mental condition that prevents obtaining informed consent is a necessary characteristic of the research population. The specific reasons for involving research subjects with a condition that renders them unable to give informed consent should be stated in the experimental protocol for consideration and approval of the review committee. The protocol should state that consent to remain in the research should be obtained as soon as possible from the individual or a legally authorized surrogate.

27. Both authors and publishers have ethical obligations. In publication of the results of research, the investigators are obliged to preserve the accuracy of the results. Negative as well as positive results should be published or otherwise publicly available. Sources of funding, institutional affiliations and any possible conflicts of interest should be declared in the publication. Reports of experimentation not in accordance with the principles laid down in this Declaration should not be accepted for publication.

C. Additional Principles for Medical Research Combined with Medical Care

28. The physician may combine medical research with medical care, only to the extent that the research is justified by its potential prophylactic, diagnostic or therapeutic value. When medical research is combined with medical care, additional standards apply to protect the patients who are research subjects.

29. The benefits, risks, burdens and effectiveness of a new method should be tested against those of the best current prophylactic, diagnostic, and therapeutic methods. This does not exclude the use of placebo, or no treatment, in studies where no proven prophylactic, diagnostic or therapeutic method exists.

30. At the conclusion of the study, every patient entered into the study should be assured of access to the best proven prophylactic, diagnostic and therapeutic methods identified by the study.

31. The physician should fully inform the patient which aspects of the care are related to the research. The refusal of a patient to participate in a study must never interfere with the patient-physician relationship.

32. In the treatment of a patient, where proven prophylactic, diagnostic and therapeutic methods do not exist or have been ineffective, the physician, with informed consent from the patient, must be free to use unproven or new prophylactic, diagnostic and therapeutic measures, if in the physician's judgement it offers hope of saving life, re-establishing health or alleviating suffering. Where possible, these measures should be made the object of research, designed to evaluate their safety and efficacy. In all cases, new information should be recorded and, where appropriate, published. The other relevant guidelines of this Declaration should be followed.

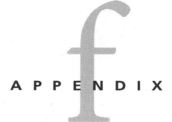

A P P E N D I X

Form FDA 1572

DEPARTMENT OF HEALTH AND HUMAN SERVICES PUBLIC HEALTH SERVICE FOOD AND DRUG ADMINISTRATION **STATEMENT OF INVESTIGATOR** *TITLE 21, CODE OF FEDERAL REGULATIONS (CFR) Part 312* (See instructions on reverse side.)	Form Approved: OMB No. 0910-004 Expiration Date: June 30, 1992 *See OMB Statement on Reverse.* Note: No investigator may participate in an investigation until her/she provides the sponsor with a completed, signed Statement of investigator. Form FDA 1572 (21 CFR 312.53)).

1. NAME AND ADDRESS OF INVESTIGATOR.

2. EDUCATION, TRAINING AND EXPERIENCE THAT QUALIFIES THE INVESTIGATOR AS AN EXPERT IN THE CLINICAL INVESTIGATION OF THE DRUG FOR TH USE UNDER INVESTIGATION. ONE OF THE FOLLOWING IS ATTACHED:

☐ CURRICULUM VITAE   ☐ OTHER STATEMENT OF QUALIFICATIONS

3. NAME AND ADDRESS OF ANY MEDICAL SCHOOL, HOSPITAL OR OTHER RESEARCH FACILITY WHERE THE CLINICAL INVESTIGATION(S) WILL BE CONDUCTED.

4. NAME AND ADDRESS OF ANY CLINICAL LABORATORY FACILITIES TO BE USED IN THE STUDY.

5. NAME AND ADDRESS OF THE INSTITUTIONAL REVIEW BOARD (IRB) THAT IS RESPONSIBLE FOR REVIEW AND APPROVAL OF THE STUDY(IES).

6. NAME(S) OF THE SUBINVESTIGATORS (e.g. research fellows, residents, associates) WHO WILL BE ASSISTING THE INVESTIGATOR IN THE CONDUCT OF THE INVESTIGATION(S).

7. NAME AND CODE NUMBER, IF ANY, OF THE PROTOCOL(S) IN THE IND FOR THE STUDY(IES) TO BE CONDUCTED BY THE INVESTIGATOR.

FORM FDA 1572 (12/91)   PREVIOUS EDITION IS OBSOLETE.

Form FDA 1572 (continued)

8. ATTACH THE FOLLOWING CLINICAL PROTOCOL INFORMATION:

☐ FOR PHASE 1 INVESTIGATIONS, A GENERAL OUTLINE OF THE PLANNED INVESTIGATION INCLUDING THE ESTIMATED DURATION OF THE STUDY AND THE MAXIMUM NUMBER OF SUBJECTS THAT WILL BE INVOLVED.

☐ FOR PHASE 2 OR 3 INVESTIGATIONS, AN OUTLINE OF THE STUDY PROTOCOL INCLUDING AN APPROXIMATION OF THE NUMBER OF SUBJECTS TO BE TREATED WITH THE DRUG AND THE NUMBER TO BE EMPLOYED AS CONTROLS IF ANY: THE CLINICAL USES TO BE INVESTIGATED: CHARACTERISTICS OF SUBJECTS BY AGE, SEX AND CONDITION; THE KIND OF CLINICAL OBSERVATIONS AND LABORATORY TESTS TO BE CONDUCTED: THE ESTIMATED DURATION OF THE STUDY; AND COPIES OR A DESCRIPTION OF CASE REPORT FORMS TO BE USED.

9. COMMITMENTS:

I agree to conduct the study(ies) in accordance with the relevant, current protocol(s) and will only make changes in a protocol after notifying the sponsor, except when necessary to protect the safety, rights, or welfare of subjects.

I agree to personally conduct or supervise the described investigation(s).

I agree to inform any patients, or any persons used as controls, that the drugs are being used for investigational purposes and I will ensure that the requirements relating to obtaining informed consent in 21 CFR Part 50 and institutional review board (IRB) review and approval in 21 CFR Part 56 are met.

I agree to report to the sponsor adverse experiences that occur in the course of the investigation(s) in accordance with 21 CFR 312.64.

I have read and understand the information in the investigator's brochure, including the potential risks and side effects of the drug.

I agree to ensure that all associates, colleagues, and employees assisting in the conduct of the study(ies) are informed about their obligations in meeting the above commitments.

I agree to maintain adequate and accurate records in accordance with 21 CFR 312 62 and to make those records available for inspection in accordance with 21 CFR 312 68.

I will ensure that an IRB that complies with the requirements of 21 CFR Part 56 will be responsible for the initial and continuing review and approval of the clinical investigation. I also agree to promptly report to the IRB all changes in the research activity and all unanticipated problems involving risks to human subjects or others. Additionally, I will not make any changes in the research without IRB approval, except where necessary to eliminate apparent immediate hazards to human subjects.

I agree to comply with all other requirements regarding the obligations of clinical investigators and all other pertinent requirements in 21 CFR Part 312.

INSTRUCTIONS FOR COMPLETING FORM FDA 1572
STATEMENT OF INVESTIGATOR:

1. Complete all sections. Attach a separate page if additional space is needed.

2. Attach curriculum vitae or other statement of qualifications as described in Section 2.

3. Attach protocol outline as described in Section 8.

4. Sign and date below.

5. FORWARD THE COMPLETED FORM AND ATTACHMENTS TO THE SPONSOR. The sponsor will incorporate this information along with other technical data into an Investigational New Drug Application (IND). INVESTIGATORS SHOULD NOT SEND THIS FORM DIRECTLY TO THE FOOD AND DRUG ADMINISTRATION.

10. SIGNATURE OF INVESTIGATOR	11. DATE

Informed Consent Form (Example)

Patient's Initials ....

<u>DRUG NAME</u>   Protocol # ....

Title: "Effects of DRUG Compared to VERAPAMIL SR on the Quality of Life and Hemodynamics in Elderly Hypertensive Patients"

I agree to participate in the clinical testing of an investigational new drug <u>DRUG</u>, which will be used in 20-mg and 40-mg doses. The 40-mg dose will be used only if my blood pressure is not controlled by the 20-mg dose. This drug will be compared to VERAPAMIL SR, a drug that has been approved for use in the United States for the treatment of high blood pressure. VERAPAMIL SR will also be used in two doses: 240 mg and 480 mg daily. The 480-mg dose will be given as 240 mg twice daily only if blood pressure is not controlled by the 240-mg once-daily dose. I understand that the study is a research project sponsored by <u>SPONSOR</u> and the <u>DRUG</u> is an experimental drug not yet approved for sale in the United States. I am between 60 and 80 years of age. I understand that the following information is provided for my benefit, and I must clearly understand it before signing my name to the final page.

Patient's Initials ....

The Nature and Purpose of this Study:

<u>DRUG</u> is a drug developed by <u>SPONSOR</u>. It belongs to a class of drugs called angiotensin-converting enzyme inhibitors, which work by blocking a substance released by the kidney that causes the small arteries in the body to constrict. This type of drug has proven useful in the treatment of high blood pressure.

VERAPAMIL SR is a medication that is a calcium channel blocker. This type of medication has proved useful in the treatment of heart disease and high blood pressure. It works by blocking the intake of calcium into the muscle cells in the small and medium-sized arteries in the body. This action causes the muscles to relax thereby allowing the arteries to dilate and blood pressure to be reduced.

The purpose of this study is to compare and evaluate the safety, tolerability and effectiveness of once-daily <u>DRUG</u> (in the two doses previously mentioned) to twice-daily VERAPAMIL SR (in a once- or twice-daily dose of 240 mg) on the control of blood pressure and the effects on the quality of life in elderly patients.

This study is part of a larger study being conducted at 10 centers throughout the United States. There will be approximately 300 patients participating.

Procedures:

In order to participate in this study I must have hypertension. If female, I must be either surgically sterile (hysterectomy or tubal ligation) or post-menopausal (one year since my last menstrual period).

I understand that there is a four-week period that occurs during this study where I will be taking a placebo (inactive substance). If, during this period, or any other part of this study, my blood pressure goes up to levels that my doctor considers dangerous, my participation in the program will be stopped and I will be placed on blood pressure medication. The side effects of these medications will be explained to me by my doctor.

After the 12th week of this study, if my blood pressure is not adequately controlled, the dosage of my medication will be increased to the higher dose of either of the medications I have been placed on. I understand that this program is conducted under "double blind" conditions, so that neither the doctor nor I will know which medication I am taking. However, if an emergency arises, that information will be available to the physician.

I understand that my participation in this study will be for 28 to 30 weeks. I will come to the clinic 10 or 11 times in this period.

I understand that I will have three electrocardiograms and five blood tests done during this study. The total amount of blood taken will be about five ounces (10 tablespoons).

I understand that for my own protection I will reveal my entire medical history. I will have a complete physical examination twice and a brief phys-

Patient's Initials ....

ical three times. I also understand that my blood pressure, heart rate and body weight will be recorded at each visit. I agree to participate in a "Quality of Life" survey five times during this program. If I decide that I no longer wish to participate at any time during this program I will be strongly encouraged to undergo an evaluation which includes a complete physical examination and laboratory safety tests (blood and urine samples). Then, I will resume my usual blood pressure medication(s).

Risk:

I understand that I will be asked to stop any blood pressure medication that I may be currently taking, which may lead to a rise in my blood pressure. There is the further risk that during the entire study my blood pressure may rise or not be adequately controlled. However, my doctor will watch my blood pressure closely. If my blood pressure goes to a level that is considered dangerous, I will be placed on other medication to control it, and the study will be immediately terminated.

Side effects seen with <u>DRUG</u> are in general similar to those seen with other ACE inhibitors. They include nausea, dizziness, rash/itching, muscle spasm, weakness, gastrointestinal disturbances, headache, lowering of white blood cell count, changes in urine protein, coughing, wheezing, shortness of breath and excessive reduction in blood pressure.

Side effects seen with VERAPAMIL SR have thus far been infrequent and usually transient. These include headache, rash, fatigue, swelling of legs, dizziness, nausea, constipation and weakness. Excessive reductions in blood pressure have also occurred rarely.

As with any drug, there may be other side effects and risks that are currently unforeseeable. If I develop any intolerable side effects, my study doctor will stop the study drug and I will be withdrawn from the study and placed on another medication.

Possible side effects from blood drawing include faintness, inflammation of the vein, pain, bruising, or bleeding at the site of venipuncture. There is also a slight possibility of infection.

Benefits:

The potential benefits I may receive from participating in this study include the close evaluation of my high blood pressure and the knowledge that the results of this study may contribute to information about a new drug to treat high blood pressure. There will be no charge to me for the medications, clinic visits, electrocardiograms and laboratory tests required by this study. No therapeutic benefit however can be guaranteed. I will receive $120 at the completion of this program to help defray my travel expenses. If I am unable to complete this program despite my good efforts to do so, I will receive $10 for each visit I have made to the clinic instead of the full $120 stipend.

Patient's Initials ....

Alternate Therapy:
Many other medications are currently available to treat high blood pressure. These medications include water pills. Other medications act to decrease the pumping activity of the heart, or cause dilation of the blood vessels in the body. Thus, it is not necessary for me to participate in this study to have my high blood pressure treated. If I decide not to participate, the study physician will help arrange medical treatment for my high blood pressure. I may stop my participation in this study at any time without penalty or loss of benefits. Representatives of SPONSOR and the study physicians may stop my participation in this study at any time without regard to my consent, if it is felt to be appropriate or in my best interest or for reasons that include, but are not limited to noncompliance with the protocol or repeated failure to keep my appointment.

I agree not to allow this medication to be taken by anyone other than myself and to keep it out of the reach of children.

Payment or medical Treatment for Injury and Source of Additional Information:

Every effort to prevent any injury that could result from this study will be taken by DOCTOR. SPONSOR will provide payment for reasonable medical expenses to treat any injury that occurs as a direct result of the drug or its proper administration that is not covered by my medical insurance. Further information on this study and information in regard to payment or medical treatment due to injury can be obtained from DOCTOR. Any such information should be reported to DOCTOR.

Authorization to Allow Inspection
of Medical Records:
It is important to SPONSOR, the U.S. Food and Drug Administration and the Institutional Review Board to be able to inspect my medical records. Therefore, I am requested to authorize my doctor to release my medical records to SPONSOR, the FDA, and the IRB. These records will be utilized by SPONSOR, the FDA, or the IRB only in connection with this study, and they will not be used for any other purpose or be disclosed to any other party without my permission. Every effort will be made by all parties involved to maintain the confidentiality of these records.

Other Considerations:
If, during the course of this study, significant new information becomes available that may relate to my willingness to continue to participate in this study, this information will be provided to me by DOCTOR and/or his/her associates.

If at any time I have any questions regarding this research or my participation, I should contact the DOCTOR at DOCTOR'S PHONE # who will answer the questions to the best of his/her ability. If I have any questions

Patient's Initials ....

regarding the study or my rights as a research subject, I should contact IRB <u>CHAIRPERSON</u> at <u>IRB CHAIRPERSON PHONE # & ADDRESS</u>. If I experience any side effects or medical problems, I should contact <u>DOCTOR</u> at <u>DOCTOR'S PHONE #</u>.

Consent:

I voluntarily consent to participate in this study with the understanding of the above mentioned risks. I also understand that I may withdraw from the study at any time whether or not it has been completed, without affecting my present or future medical care at <u>DOCTOR'S OFFICE</u>.

I understand that refusal to participate will involve no penalty or loss of benefits to which I am entitled. I have read and understand the preceding information describing the study. All my questions have been answered to my satisfaction and this form is being signed voluntarily indicating my desire to participate in this study. My signature below acknowledges that I have been given a copy of this form for my personal records.

Subject's signature .... Initials .... Date ....

Witness signature .... Date ....

Physician's signature .... Date ....

h

Financial Disclosure by Clinical Investigators

U.S. Department of Health and Human Services
Food and Drug Administration
Center for Drug Evaluation and Research
Center for Biologics Evaluation and Research
Center for Devices and Radiological Health
March 20, 2001

Guidance for Industry

Financial Disclosure by Clinical Investigators

This guidance represents the Food and Drug Administration's current thinking on this topic. It does not create or confer any rights for or on any person and does not operate to bind FDA or the public. An alternative approach may be used if such approach satisfies the requirements of the applicable statute, regulations, or both.

I. Introduction

On February 2, 1998, FDA published a final rule requiring anyone who submits a marketing application of any drug, biological product or device to submit certain information concerning the compensation to, and financial interests of, any clinical investigator conducting clinical studies covered by the rule. This requirement, which became effective on February 2, 1999, applies to any clinical study submitted in a marketing application that the applicant or FDA relies on to establish that the product is effective, and any study in which a single investigator makes a significant contribution to the demonstration of safety. This final rule requires applicants to certify to the absence of certain financial interests of clinical investigators or to disclose those financial interests. If the applicant does not include certification and/or disclosure, or does not certify that it was not possible to obtain the information, the agency may refuse to file the application. On December 31, 1998, FDA published an amended final rule that reduced the need to gather certain financial information for studies completed before February 2, 1999. On October 26, 1999, FDA published a draft guidance to provide clarification in interpreting and complying with these regulations. The burden hours required for Section 21 CFR Part 54 are reported and approved under OMB Control Number 0910 0396.

II. Financial Disclosure Requirements

Under the applicable regulations (21 CFR Parts 54, 312, 314, 320, 330, 601, 807, 812, 814, and 860), an applicant is required to submit to FDA a list of clinical investigators who conducted covered clinical studies and certify and/or disclose certain financial arrangements as follows:
1. Certification that no financial arrangements with an investigator have been made where study outcome could affect compensation; that the investigator has no proprietary interest in the tested product; that the investigator does not have a significant equity interest in the sponsor of the covered study; and that the investigator has not received significant payments of other sorts; and/or
2. Disclosure of specified financial arrangements and any steps taken to minimize the potential for bias.

Disclosable Financial Arrangements:
A. Compensation made to the investigator in which the value of compensation could be affected by study outcome. This requirement applies to all covered studies, whether ongoing or completed as of February 2, 1999.
B. A proprietary interest in the tested product, including, but not limited to, a patent, trademark, copyright or licensing agreement. This requirement applies to all covered studies, whether ongoing or completed as of February 2, 1999.

C. Any equity interest in the sponsor of a covered study, i.e., any ownership interest, stock options, or other financial interest whose value cannot be readily determined through reference to public prices. This requirement applies to all covered studies, whether ongoing or completed;

D. Any equity interest in a publicly held company that exceeds $50,000 in value. These must be disclosed only for covered clinical studies that are ongoing on or after February 2, 1999. The requirement applies to interests held during the time the clinical investigator is carrying out the study and for 1 year following completion of the study; and

E. Significant payments of other sorts, which are payments that have a cumulative monetary value of $25,000 or more made by the sponsor of a covered study to the investigator or the investigators' institution to support activities of the investigator exclusive of the costs of conducting the clinical study or other clinical studies, (e.g., a grant to fund ongoing research, compensation in the form of equipment or retainers for ongoing consultation or honoraria) during the time the clinical investigator is carrying out the study and for 1 year following completion of the study. This requirement applies to payments made on or after February 2, 1999.

Agency Actions

If FDA determines that the financial interests of any clinical investigator raise a serious question about the integrity of the data, FDA will take any action it deems necessary to ensure the reliability of the data including:

- Initiating agency audits of the data derived from the clinical investigator in question;
- Requesting that the applicant submit further analyses of data, e.g., to evaluate the effect of the clinical investigator's data on the overall study outcome;
- Requesting that the applicant conduct additional independent studies to confirm the results of the questioned study; and
- Refusing to treat the covered clinical study as providing data that can be the basis for an agency action.

Definitions

- *Clinical Investigator* – means any listed or identified investigator or subinvestigator who is directly involved in the treatment or evaluation of research subjects. The term also includes the spouse and each dependent child of the investigator.
- *Covered clinical study* – means any study of a drug, biological product or device in humans submitted in a marketing application or reclassification petition that the applicant or FDA relies on to establish that the product is effective (including studies that show equivalence to an effective product) or any study in which a single investigator makes a significant contribution to the demonstration of safety. This would, in general, not include phase 1 tolerance studies or pharmacokinetic

studies, most clinical pharmacology studies (unless they are critical to an efficacy determination), large open safety studies conducted at multiple sites, treatment protocols and parallel track protocols. An applicant may consult with FDA as to which clinical studies constitute "covered clinical studies" for purposes of complying with financial disclosure requirements.

- *Applicant* – means the party who submits a marketing application to FDA for approval of a drug, device or biologic product or who submits a reclassification petition. The applicant is responsible for submitting the required certification and disclosure statements.

- *Sponsor of the covered clinical study* – means the party providing support for a particular study at the time it was carried out.

III. PURPOSE

The financial disclosure regulations were intended to ensure that financial interests and arrangements of clinical investigators that could affect the reliability of data submitted to FDA are identified and disclosed by the applicant. FDA has received many questions concerning the implementation of this final rule. The agency is issuing this guidance to respond to these questions. FDA encourages applicants and sponsors to contact the agency for advice concerning specific circumstances that may raise concerns as early in the product development process as possible.

IV. QUESTIONS AND ANSWERS

Q. Why did FDA develop financial disclosure regulations?

A: In June 1991, the Inspector General of the Department of Health and Human Services submitted a management advisory report to FDA stating that FDA's failure to have a mechanism for collecting information on "financial conflicts of interest" of clinical investigators who study products that undergo FDA review could constitute a material weakness under the Federal Manager's Financial Integrity Act. Although FDA determined that a material weakness did not exist, the agency did conclude that there was a need to address this issue through rulemaking. During the rulemaking process, FDA also learned about potentially problematic financial arrangements through published newspaper articles, Congressional inquiries, public testimony, and comments. Based on the information gathered, FDA determined that it was appropriate to require the submission of certain financial information with marketing applications that include certain types of clinical data.

Q: Are applicants required to use FDA forms 3454 and 3455 in reporting this information?

A: Yes. The regulations require that the applicant submit one completed Form 3454 for all clinical investigators certifying to the absence of financial interests and arrangements. The applicant may append a list of investigator names to Form 3454 for those investigators certifying that those investigators hold none of the identifiable disclosable financial arrangements. For any clinical investigator for whom the applicant does not submit the certification, the applicant must submit a completed Form 3455 disclosing the financial interests and arrangements and steps taken to minimize the potential for bias.

Where an applicant cannot provide a blanket certification for all investigators because of the existence of disclosable financial arrangements for one or more investigators, an applicant should complete a disclosure form 3455 for each investigator having disclosable financial arrangements. The applicant should identify the specific covered clinical study (or studies) at issue and provide detailed information about the specific relationship that is being disclosed, (e.g., the nature of the contingent payment or the equity holdings of the investigator or the investigator's spouse or dependent child that exceeded the threshold). This disclosure needs to be linked to the specific covered clinical study (or studies) in which the investigators participated.

In those instances where the applicant cannot provide complete certification or disclosure on all arrangements (e.g., the applicant has information about 2 of the 4 requirements but has been unable to obtain the rest of the information), the applicant should certify that despite the applicant's due diligence in attempting to obtain the information, the applicant was unable to obtain the information and should include an explanation of how the applicant attempted to obtain the information and why the information was not obtainable.

Q: What does FDA mean by the term "due diligence"?

A: "Due diligence" is a measure of activity expected from a reasonable and prudent person under a particular circumstance. In complying with these rules, sponsors and applicants should use reasonable judgement in deciding how much effort needs to be expended to collect this information. If sponsors/applicants find it impossible to obtain the financial information in question, applicants should explain why this information was not obtainable and document attempts made in an effort to collect the information.

Q: Who, specifically, is responsible for signing the financial certification/disclosure forms?

A: The forms are to be signed and dated by a responsible corporate official or representative of the applicant (e.g., the chief financial officer).

Q. Where in a drug/biologic application should an applicant include certification that financial arrangements of concern do not exist or the disclosure of those arrangements that do exist? Where should the information be included in a device application?

A: For drugs and biological product applications, applicants should include the financial certification/disclosure forms as part of item 19 (other) of the application. See form 356h. FDA is revising the current form 356h and upon completion of this revision, financial certification and disclosure information will become number 19 and (other) will become number 20. For device applications, applicants should submit the financial certification/disclosure forms according to the format outlined in the appropriate submission checklist.

Q: What obligations do IND and IDE sponsors have regarding information collection prior to study start?

A: The regulations, 21 CFR 312.53 and 21 CFR 812.43, provide that before permitting an investigator to begin participation in an investigation, the IND/IDE sponsor shall obtain sufficient accurate financial information that will allow an applicant to submit complete and accurate certification or disclosure statements required under Part 54. The sponsor is also required to obtain the investigator's commitment to promptly update this information if any relevant changes occur during the course of the investigation and for one year following completion of the study. By collecting the information prior to study start, the sponsor will be aware of any potential problems, can consult with the agency early on, and take steps to minimize the potential for bias. See question and answer 7 for additional information.

Q: What is the responsibility of the IND/IDE sponsor for obtaining financial information from investigators at the IND/IDE stage when the IND/IDE sponsor is not the party who will be submitting a marketing application?

A: The term "sponsor" has somewhat different meanings in the regulations at 312.53/812.43 and 54.2. An applicant must report financial interests in the sponsor of the covered study. Under 21 CFR 54.2, "sponsor" is defined as the party "supporting a particular study at the time it was carried out." FDA interprets support to include those who provide "material support",e.g., monetary support or test product under study. The sponsor of an IND or IDE, as defined in 21 CFR 312 and 812 is the "party or parties who take responsibility for and initiate a clinical investigation". The term "sponsor" is also used in 312.53 and 812.43 to refer to the party who will be submitting a marketing application (who is also responsible for submitting the certification and disclosure statement required by Part 54).

In most cases, the IND/IDE sponsor, the sponsor of the covered study, and the applicant company are the same party, but there are times where they may be different. For example, when an academic or government institution or CRO conducts a covered study and is the IND/IDE sponsor (Part 312/812 sponsor), a drug or device company that provides funding or the test article used in the study is a Part 54 sponsor, and is likely to be the applicant if a marketing application is submitted to FDA. If the drug or device company that was a sponsor of the covered study sold the drug/device to another company, the applicant could be neither the IND/IDE sponsor nor a Part 54 sponsor.

The responsibility for reporting financial information to FDA falls upon the applicant; that is, the final rule (Part 54) requires that the applicant company submit financial information on clinical investigators at the time the marketing application is submitted to the agency. The information that the applicant must report, apart from compensation that may be affected by study outcome and proprietary interests is:

1. equity interests in a Part 54 sponsor of a covered study (e.g., any interest that cannot be valued through reference to public prices and interest in excess of $50,000 in a publicly held company), and
2. significant payments of other sorts by a Part 54 sponsor of a covered study.

Although reporting to the FDA is the responsibility of the applicant, the IND/IDE holder (part 312/812 sponsor) is required to collect the financial information before permitting an investigator to participate in a clinical study (312.53 and 812.43). The purpose of this requirement is two fold:

1. to alert the IND/IDE sponsor of the study to any potentially problematic financial interest as early in the drug development process as possible in order to minimize the potential for study bias and
2. to facilitate accurate collection of data that may be submitted many years later.

The IND/IDE sponsor, who is in contact with the investigator, is best placed to inquire as to the financial arrangements of investigators, and this obligation applies to any IND/IDE sponsor (e.g., commercial, government or CRO). The IND/IDE sponsor shall maintain complete and accurate records showing any financial interest as described in Section 54.4 (a) (3) (i-iv) in a sponsor of the covered study. The IND/IDE sponsor is responsible for ensuring that required financial information is collected and is made available to the applicant company, so that, the information can be included in the NDA/BLA/PMA submission.

Q. **The applicant is obligated to disclose financial interests related only to >covered studies, specifically those relied upon to provide support for the effectiveness of a product and certain others. An IND holder (IND sponsor), acting much earlier, must inquire into investigator financial interests before the ultimate role of a study in the application is determined. How will the IND sponsor determine which studies will ultimately require certification/disclosure statements?**

A: The IND sponsor will need to consider the potential role of a particular study based on study size, design and other considerations. Almost any controlled effectiveness study could, depending on outcome, become part of a marketing application, but other studies might be critical too, such as a pharmacodynamic study in a population subset or a bioequivalence study supporting a new dosage form.

Q. **If a Contract Research Organization (CRO) is conducting a covered clinical study on behalf of another company, should the CRO collect the financial information from investigators? Is it necessary to collect financial information from investigators who have financial interests in CROs?**

A: With regard to CRO and commercial sponsor arrangements, the same principles as articulated in answer 6 would apply. For example, if a CRO meets the definition of an IND/IDE sponsor or has contracted to collect financial information from investigators on behalf of an IND/IDE sponsor, the CRO must collect financial information on clinical investigators' interests in Part 54 sponsors (312.53, 812.43). If the CRO provides material support for a covered study, financial information on clinical investigators' interests in the CRO is to be collected. If another entity provided material support for the study, the CRO also would collect financial information relative to that entity.

Q: **Suppose a public or academic institution conducts a study without any support from a commercial sponsor, but the study is then used by an applicant to support its marketing application. In that case, who is the "sponsor" of the study and what information should the applicant submit?**

A: In this case, the Part 54 sponsor of the study is the public or academic institution. Because such institutions are not commercial entities, in many instances, there will not be relevant equity interests to report. However, any relevant interests under 54.4, such as any proprietary interest in the tested product, including but not limited to a patent, trademark, copyright or licensing agreement are to be reported.

Q: Does FDA have expectations about how the financial information should be collected? Will FDA consider it acceptable practice for a company to use a questionnaire to collect financial information from investigators rather than constructing an internal system to collect and report this information?

A: FDA has no preference as to how this information is collected from investigators. Under this rule, sponsors/applicants have the flexibility to collect the information in the most efficient and least burdensome manner that will be effective, for example, through questionnaires completed by the clinical investigators or by using information already available to the sponsor. FDA does not require sponsors to establish elaborate tracking systems to collect the information.

Q. What does FDA mean by the definition of clinical investigator and subinvestigator? Is it necessary to collect financial information on spouses and dependent children of subinvestigators?

A: The definition of "clinical investigator" in Part 54 is intended to identify the individuals who should be considered investigators for purposes of reporting under the rule, generally, the people taking responsibility for the study at a given study site. For drugs, biological products and devices, it should be noted that hospital staff, including nurses, residents, or fellows and office staff who provide ancillary or intermittent care but who do not make direct and significant contribution to the data are not meant to be included under the definition of clinical investigator. For purposes of this financial disclosure regulation, the term investigator also includes the spouse and each dependent child of the investigator and subinvestigator.

For drugs and biological products, clinical investigator means the individual(s) who actually conduct(s) and take(s) responsibility for an investigation, i.e. under whose immediate direction the drug or biologic is administered or dispensed to a subject or who is directly involved in the evaluation of research subjects. Where an investigation is directed by more than one person at a site, there may be more than one investigator who must report. For purposes of this rule, the terms investigators and subinvestigators include persons who fit any of these criteria: sign the Form FDA 1572, are identified as an investigator in initial submissions or protocol amendments under an IND, or are identified as an investigator in the NDA/BLA. For studies not conducted under an IND, the sponsor will need to identify the investigators and subinvestigators they consider covered by the rule in form 3454 and/or 3455. We expect that there will be at least one such person at each clinical site. If, however, there are other persons who are responsible for a study at a site, those persons should also be included as investigators.

For medical devices, clinical investigators are defined as individual(s), under whose immediate direction the subject is treated and the investigational device is administered, including follow-up evaluations and treatments. Where an investigation is conducted by a team of individuals, the investigator is the responsible leader of the team. In general, investigators and subinvestigators sign "investigator agreements" in accordance with 21 CFR 812.43(c) and it is these individuals whose interests should be reported. For studies not conducted under an FDA-approved IDE, (that is, a non-significant risk IDE or an exempt study), the sponsor would need to identify the investigators and subinvestigators they considered covered by the rule in form 3454 and 3455. We expect that there will be at least one such person at each site.

Q: **Do the reporting requirements apply to efficacy studies that include large numbers of investigators and multiple sites? Will the agency consider a waiver mechanism to exempt applicants from collecting information from clinical investigators conducting these kinds of studies?**

A: Large multi-center efficacy studies with many investigators are considered covered clinical studies within the meaning of the final rule. See 21 CFR 54.2(c). Data from investigators having only a small percentage of the total subject population (in a study with large numbers of investigators and multiple sites) may still affect the overall study results. For example, if a sponsor submitted data collected during a large, multi-center, double blind study that included several thousand subjects and a single clinical investigator at one of the largest sites enrolled one percent of subjects, that investigator could still be responsible for a significant number of subjects. If the investigator fabricated data or otherwise affected the integrity of the data, remaining data for the drug may not meet the statistical criteria for efficacy as defined prospectively in the protocol.

Because the regulations (see 21 CFR 312.10, 812.10, 314.90 and 814.20) allow a sponsor to seek a waiver of certain requirements, applicants may seek waivers of the financial disclosure requirements. FDA believes it is highly unlikely, however, that any waivers will be justified for studies begun after February 2, 1999, because the sponsor should already have begun collecting the information on an ongoing basis. FDA will evaluate any request for waiver on a case-by-case basis.

Q: **The rule requires that investigators provide information on financial interests during the course of the study and for one year after completion of the study (see 54.4(b))? What does "completion of the study" mean?**

A: Completion of the study means that all study subjects have been enrolled and follow up of primary endpoint data on all subjects has been completed in accordance with the clinical protocol. Many studies have more than one stage (e.g., a study could have a short term endpoint and a longer term follow up phase). Completion of the study here refers to that part of the study being submitted in the application. If there were a subsequent application based on longer term data, completion of the study would be defined similarly for the new data. It is not required that an applicant submit updated financial information to FDA after submission of the application, but applicants must retain complete records. Where there is more than one study site, the sponsor may consider completion of the study to be when the last study site is complete, or may consider each study site individually as it is completed.

Q: **Do applicant companies need to collect information for a year after completion of the study? Who is responsible for collecting/providing this information?**

A: According to the February 2, 1998 final rule, the investigator must provide updated information when the investigator holds any equity interest in a privately held company or if stock holdings in a publicly held company exceed $50,000 in value during the one year period following completion of the study. In addition, sponsors/applicants must keep records on file when significant payments of other sorts are paid by the sponsor of the covered study to the investigator or the investigator's institution to support activities of the investigator that have a cumulative monetary value of more than $25,000, exclusive of the costs of conducting the covered clinical studies, during the study and for one year following completion of the study. FDA specified the one-year time frame because anticipation of payments may be as influential as payments already received. Applicants need only report on these arrangements when the marketing application is submitted, but sponsors/applicants are responsible for keeping updated financial information from the investigators in company files.

Q: **What information about a financial interest should be disclosed to the agency? For example, if an investigator owns more than $50,000 of stock in a publicly held company, can the applicant just disclose that there is an interest that exceeds the $50,000 threshold or is it necessary to disclose in written detail the arrangement in question?**

A: The applicant must disclose specific details of the financial interest including the size and nature of the financial interest in question and any steps taken to minimize the potential for study bias that such an interest represents.

Q: Is the clinical investigator required to report all fluctuations above and below the $50,000 level during the course of the investigation and one year after completion of the study?

A: The rule requires sponsors/applicants to obtain financial information from clinical investigators and a commitment from clinical investigators to promptly update financial information, if any relevant changes occur during the course of the covered clinical study and for one year following the completion of the study [21 CFR 312.53(c)(4), 312.64(d), 812.43(c)(5), 812.110(d)]. In light of the potential volatility of stock prices, FDA recognizes that the dollar value of an investigator's equity holding in a sponsoring/applicant company is likely to fluctuate during the course of a trial. Clinical investigators should report an equity interest when the investigator becomes aware that the holding has exceeded the threshold and the investigator should use judgement in updating and reporting on fluctuations in equity interests exceeding $50,000. FDA does not expect the investigator to report when that equity interest fluctuates below that threshold.

Q. Are equity interests in mutual funds and 401K(s) reportable?

A: Because an investigator would not have control over buying or selling stocks in mutual funds, these would not be reportable. In most circumstances, interests in 401K(s) would not be reportable, although equity interest in a product over $50,000 would be reportable if it is a holding in a self directed 401K.

Q: Does the rule include ANDAs? Does the rule include 510(k)s that do not include clinical data?

A: The rule applies to any clinical study of a drug (including a biological product) or device submitted in a marketing application that the applicant or FDA relies on to establish that the product is effective, including studies of drugs that show equivalence to an approved product. This means that ANDAs are covered by the final rule. 510(k)s that do not include clinical data would not contain covered studies and therefore, no financial information from device manufacturers is needed for those applications.

Q: Do applicants need to provide information on investigators who participate in foreign studies?

A: Yes, applicants should include either a certification or disclosure of information for investigators participating in foreign covered studies. Where the applicant is unable to obtain the information despite acting with due diligence, the applicant may submit a statement documenting its efforts to obtain the information. In this case, it is unnecessary to submit a certification or disclosure form.

Q: Does the rule apply to studies in support of labeling changes?

A: The rule applies to studies submitted in a supplement when those studies meet the definition of a covered clinical study. It also applies to studies to support safety labeling changes where individual investigators make a significant contribution to the safety information.

Q: In the case where a subsidiary company of a larger parent company is conducting a covered clinical trial, is the applicant (subsidiary company) required to report information from clinical investigators about financial interests in only the subsidiary company, or is the applicant also required to report financial holdings, if any, of the investigator in the larger parent company?

A: If the subsidiary company meets the definition of sponsor of the covered study as defined under Part 54, the IND/IDE holder is required to collect from clinical investigators financial information related to the subsidiary company. The IND/IDE holder also must collect financial information related to the parent company if the parent company is a Part 54 sponsor of the study in question. If there are multiple companies providing material support for a covered study, the IND/IDE holder is responsible for collecting financial information from clinical investigators related to all companies providing that support. The applicant company is ultimately responsible for submitting financial information to the Agency at the time the marketing application is submitted.

Q: Do "actual use studies" to support a request to switch a drug product from prescription to over-the-counter (OTC) status fit the definition of covered clinical study?

A: Applicants who file supplements requesting that FDA approve a switch of a prescription drug to OTC status or who file a new drug application for direct OTC use often conduct "actual use studies." These may be intended to demonstrate that the product is safe and effective when used without the supervision of a licensed practitioner; in other cases, they may test labeling comprehension or other aspects of treatment. Actual use studies performed to support these applications would be considered covered clinical studies if they were used to demonstrate effectiveness in the OTC setting or if it is a safety study where any investigator makes a significant contribution.

Q: Are clinical investigators of in vitro diagnostics (IVDs) covered under this regulation since they often involve specimens, not human subjects?

A: Yes. Applicants who submit marketing applications for IVDs must include the appropriate financial certification or disclosure information. Under section 21 CFR 812.3(p), "subject" is defined as a "human who participates in an investigation, either as an individual on whom or on whose specimen an investigational device is used or as a control." Thus, an investigation of an IVD is considered a clinical investigation and, if it is used to support a marketing application, it would be subject to this regulation.

Q: How do significant payments of other sorts (SPOOS) relate to the variety of payments the sponsor might make to an individual or institution for various activities?

A: The term "significant payments of other sorts" was intended to capture substantial payments or other support provided to an investigator that could create a sense of obligation to the sponsor.

These payments do not include payments for the conduct of the clinical trial of the product under consideration or clinical trials of other products, under a contractual arrangement, but do include other payments made directly to the investigator or to an institution for direct support of the investigator. These payments would include honoraria, consulting fees, grant support for laboratory activities and equipment or actual equipment for the laboratory/clinic. This means that if an investigator were given equipment or money to purchase equipment for use in the laboratory/clinic, but not in relation to the conduct of the clinical trial, the payment would be considered a significant payment of other sorts and should be reported. If however, the investigator were provided with computer software or money to buy the software needed for use in the clinical trial, that would not need to be reported. Finally, payments made to the institution or to other nonstudy participating investigators that are not made on behalf of the investigator do not need to be reported.

Q: Are payments made to investigators to cover travel expenses (such as transportation, lodgings and meal expenses) trackable under significant payments of other sorts (SPOOS)?

A: Generally, reasonable payments made to investigators to cover reimbursable expenses such as transportation, lodgings and meals do not fall within the purview of SPOOS and, therefore, would not need to be tracked. Travel costs associated with transporting, providing lodgings and meals for family members of investigators are considered unnecessary and should be tracked as SPOOS. In addition, other payments that exceed reasonable expectations, (for example, an investigator is flown to a resort location for an extra week of vacation) are considered outside of normal reimbursable expenditures and are not considered expenses that are necessary to conduct the study. Therefore, these types of expenses are also reportable and should be tracked as SPOOS.

Q: Under what circumstances would FDA refuse to file an application?

A: FDA may refuse to file any marketing application that does not contain either a certification that no specified financial arrangement exists or a disclosure statement identifying the specified arrangements or a statement that the applicant has acted with due diligence to obtain the required information, and an explanation of why it was unable to do so. The agency does not anticipate that it will be necessary to use its refuse to file authority often in the context of this financial disclosure rule. Applicants are encouraged to discuss their concerns on particular matters about financial information with FDA.

Q: Who will review a disclosure of the specified financial arrangements when such information is submitted in a marketing application? How will the financial information be handled during the review of the application?

A: Applicants are required to disclose specified financial information and any steps taken to minimize the potential for bias in any drug, biological product or device marketing application submitted to the agency on or after February 2, 1999. (See 21 CFR 54.4(a)(3)). FDA review staff, including project managers, consumer safety officers, medical officers and others in the supervisory chain will review this information on a case-by-case basis.

Q: Under what circumstances will FDA publicly discuss financial arrangements disclosed to the agency?

A: In the preamble to the final rule, FDA stated that certain types of financial information requested under the rule, notably clinical investigators' equity interests would be protected from public disclosure unless circumstances relating to the public interest clearly outweigh the clinical investigator's identified privacy interest. FDA cited the example of a financial arrangement so affecting the reliability of a study as to warrant its public disclosure during evaluation of the study by an advisory panel. FDA expects that only rarely would an investigator's privacy interest be outweighed by the public interest and thus warrant disclosure of the financial interest. It is difficult to predict all possible situations that may result in public disclosure of financial interests of a clinical investigator.

The agency will carefully evaluate each circumstance on a case-by-case basis.

Q: Can FDA have access to documents related to financial disclosure or certification documents during an inspection?

A: Yes, FDA has the authority to have access to and to copy documents supporting an applicant's certification or disclosure statement submitted to the agency in a marketing application. Regulations implementing sections 505(i), 519, and 520(g) of the Act require sponsors to establish and maintain records of data (including but not limited to analytical reports by investigators) obtained during investigational studies of drugs, biological products, and devices, that will enable the Secretary to evaluate a product's safety and effectiveness. Under 54.6, applicants must retain certain information on clinical investigators' financial interests and permits FDA employees to have access to and copy them at reasonable times.

Q: What kind of documentation is necessary for manufacturers to keep in case questions about certification and/or disclosure arise?

A: To the extent that applicants have relied on investigators as the source of information about potentially disclosable financial interests in any of the four categories, the underlying documentation – e.g., copies of executed questionnaires returned by investigators , correspondence on the subject of financial disclosure, mail receipts, etc. should be retained. Likewise, to the extent that applicants who did not sponsor a covered clinical study rely on information furnished by the sponsor, the underlying documentation, including all relevant correspondence with and reports from the sponsor should be retained. To the extent that applicants rely upon information available internally, all appropriate financial documentation regarding the financial interests or arrangements in question should be retained. For example, in the case of "significant payments of other sorts," sponsors should keep documentation including, but not limited to, check stubs, canceled checks, records of electronic financial transactions, certified mail deliver receipts, etc.

Q: Where are forms FDA 3454 and 3455 located on the Web?

A: The forms are located at the following Internet address:
http://www.fda.gov/opacom/morechoices/fdaforms/cder.html

Q: Who are the contact persons in each FDA Center to answer questions during this implementation phase?

A: The following persons may be contacted: Ms. Linda Carter in the Center for Drug Evaluation and Research, phone (301) 594-6758, Dr. Joanne Less in the Center for Devices and Radiological Health, phone (301) 594-1190, and Dr. Jerome Donlon in the Center for Biologics Evaluation and Research, phone (301) 827-3028.

---

[1] This guidance has been prepared by the Implementation Team for Financial Disclosure comprised of individuals in the Office of the Commissioner, the Center for Drug Evaluation and Research (CDER), Center Biologics Evaluation and Research (CBER) and Center Devices and Radiological Health (CDRH) at the Food and Drug Administration.

APPENDIX h

Code of Federal Regulations

TITLE 21 – FOOD AND DRUGS

Chapter I – Food and Drug Administration, Department of Health and Human Services

Part 50 – Protection of Human Subjects
Part 54 – Financial Disclosure by Clinical Investigators
Part 56 – Institutional Review Boards
Part 312 – Investigational New Drug Application

Part 50

Protection of Human Subjects

Subpart A – General Provisions

Sec. 50.1 Scope.

a. This part applies to all clinical investigations regulated by the Food and Drug Administration under sections 505(i), 507(d), and 520(g) of the Federal Food, Drug, and Cosmetic Act, as well as clinical investigations that support applications for research or marketing permits for products regulated by the Food and Drug Administration, including food and color additives, drugs for human use, medical devices for human use, biological products for human use, and electronic products. Additional specific obligations and commitments of, and standards of conduct for, persons who sponsor or monitor clinical investigations involving particular test articles may also be found in other parts (e.g., parts 312 and 812). Compliance with these parts is intended to protect the rights and safety of subjects involved in investigations filed with the Food and Drug Administration pursuant to sections 406, 409, 502, 503, 505, 506, 507, 510, 513-516, 518-520, 721, and 801 of the Federal Food, Drug, and Cosmetic Act and sections 351 and 354-360F of the Public Health Service Act.

b. References in this part to regulatory sections of the Code of Federal Regulations are to chapter I of title 21, unless otherwise noted.
   [45 FR 36390, May 30, 1980; 46 FR 8979, Jan. 27, 1981]

Sec. 50.3 Definitions.

As used in this part:

a. Act means the Federal Food, Drug, and Cosmetic Act, as amended (secs. 201 – 902, 52 Stat. 1040 et seq. as amended (21 U.S.C. 321 – 392)).

b. Application for research or marketing permit includes:

   1. A color additive petition, described in part 71.

   2. A food additive petition, described in parts 171 and 571.

   3. Data and information about a substance submitted as part of the procedures for establishing that the substance is generally recognized as safe for use that results or may reasonably be expected to result, directly or indirectly, in its becoming a component or otherwise affecting the characteristics of any food, described in Secs. 170.30 and 570.30.

   4. Data and information about a food additive submitted as part of the procedures for food additives permitted to be used on an interim basis pending additional study, described in Sec. 180.1.

   5. Data and information about a substance submitted as part of the procedures for establishing a tolerance for unavoidable contami-

nants in food and food-packaging materials, described in section 406 of the act.

6. An investigational new drug application, described in part 312 of this chapter.

7. A new drug application, described in part 314.

8. Data and information about the bioavailability or bioequivalence of drugs for human use submitted as part of the procedures for issuing, amending, or repealing a bioequivalence requirement, described in part 320.

9. Data and information about an over-the-counter drug for human use submitted as part of the procedures for classifying these drugs as generally recognized as safe and effective and not misbranded, described in part 330.

10. Data and information about a prescription drug for human use submitted as part of the procedures for classifying these drugs as generally recognized as safe and effective and not misbranded, described in this chapter.

11. Data and information about an antibiotic drug submitted as part of the procedures for issuing, amending, or repealing regulations for these drugs, described in Sec. 314.300 of this chapter.

12. An application for a biological product license, described in part 601.

13. Data and information about a biological product submitted as part of the procedures for determining that licensed biological products are safe and effective and not misbranded, described in part 601.

14. Data and information about an in vitro diagnostic product submitted as part of the procedures for establishing, amending, or repealing a standard for these products, described in part 809.

15. An Application for an Investigational Device Exemption, described in part 812.

16. Data and information about a medical device submitted as part of the procedures for classifying these devices, described in section 513.

17. Data and information about a medical device submitted as part of the procedures for establishing, amending, or repealing a standard for these devices, described in section 514.

18. An application for premarket approval of a medical device, described in section 515.

19. A product development protocol for a medical device, described in section 515.

20. Data and information about an electronic product submitted as part of the procedures for establishing, amending, or repealing a standard for these products, described in section 358 of the Public Health Service Act.

21. Data and information about an electronic product submitted as part of the procedures for obtaining a variance from any electronic product performance standard, as described in Sec. 1010.4.

22. Data and information about an electronic product submitted as part of the procedures for granting, amending, or extending an exemption from a radiation safety performance standard, as described in Sec. 1010.5.

c. Clinical investigation means any experiment that involves a test article and one or more human subjects and that either is subject to requirements for prior submission to the Food and Drug Administration under section 505(i), 507(d), or 520(g) of the act, or is not subject to requirements for prior submission to the Food and Drug Administration under these sections of the act, but the results of which are intended to be submitted later to, or held for inspection by, the Food and Drug Administration as part of an application for a research or marketing permit. The term does not include experiments that are subject to the provisions of part 58 of this chapter, regarding nonclinical laboratory studies.

d. Investigator means an individual who actually conducts a clinical investigation, i.e., under whose immediate direction the test article is administered or dispensed to, or used involving, a subject, or, in the event of an investigation conducted by a team of individuals, is the responsible leader of that team.

e. Sponsor means a person who initiates a clinical investigation, but who does not actually conduct the investigation, i.e., the test article is administered or dispensed to or used involving, a subject under the immediate direction of another individual. A person other than an individual (e.g., corporation or agency) that uses one or more of its own employees to conduct a clinical investigation it has initiated is considered to be a sponsor (not a sponsor-investigator), and the employees are considered to be investigators.

f. Sponsor-investigator means an individual who both initiates and actually conducts, alone or with others, a clinical investigation, i.e., under whose immediate direction the test article is administered or dispensed to, or used involving, a subject. The term does not include any person other than an individual, e.g., corporation or agency.

g. Human subject means an individual who is or becomes a participant in research, either as a recipient of the test article or as a control. A subject may be either a healthy human or a patient.

h. Institution means any public or private entity or agency (including Federal, State, and other agencies). The word facility as used in section 520(g) of the act is deemed to be synonymous with the term institution for purposes of this part.

i. Institutional review board (IRB) means any board, committee, or other group formally designated by an institution to review biomedical research involving humans as subjects, to approve the initiation of and conduct periodic review of such research. The term has the same meaning as the phrase institutional review committee as used in section 520(g) of the act.

j. Test article means any drug (including a biological product for human use), medical device for human use, human food additive, color additive, electronic product, or any other article subject to regulation under the act or under sections 351 and 354-360F of the Public Health Service Act (42 U.S.C. 262 and 263b-263n).

k. Minimal risk means that the probability and magnitude of harm or discomfort anticipated in the research are not greater in and of themselves than those ordinarily encountered in daily life or during the performance of routine physical or psychological examinations or tests.

l. Legally authorized representative means an individual or judicial or other body authorized under applicable law to consent on behalf of a prospective subject to the subject's particpation in the procedure(s) involved in the research.

m. Family member means any one of the following legally competent persons: Spouse; parents; children (including adopted children); brothers, sisters, and spouses of brothers and sisters; and any individual related by blood or affinity whose close association with the subject is the equivalent of a family relationship.

[45 FR 36390, May 30, 1980, as amended at 46 FR 8950, Jan. 27, 1981; 54 FR 9038, Mar. 3, 1989; 56 FR 28028, June 18, 1991; 61 FR 51528, Oct. 2, 1996; 62 FR 39440, July 23, 1997]

Subpart B – Informed Consent of Human Subjects

Sec. 50.20 General requirements for informed consent.

Source: 46 FR 8951, Jan. 27, 1981, unless otherwise noted.

Except as provided in Sec. 50.23, no investigator may involve a human being as a subject in research covered by these regulations unless the investigator has obtained the legally effective informed consent of the subject or the subject's legally authorized representative. An investigator shall seek such consent only under circumstances that provide the prospective subject or the representative sufficient opportunity to consider whether or not to participate and that minimize the possibility of coercion or undue influence. The information that is given to the subject or the representative shall be in language understandable to the subject or the representative. No informed consent, whether oral or written, may include any exculpatory language through which the subject or the representative is made to waive or appear to waive any of the subject's legal rights, or releases or appears to release the investigator, the sponsor, the institution, or its agents from liability for negligence.

Sec. 50.23 Exception from general requirements.

a. The obtaining of informed consent shall be deemed feasible unless, before use of the test article (except as provided in paragraph (b) of this section), both the investigator and a physician who is not otherwise participating in the clinical investigation certify in writing all of the following:

1. The human subject is confronted by a life-threatening situation necessitating the use of the test article.
2. Informed consent cannot be obtained from the subject because of an inability to communicate with, or obtain legally effective consent from, the subject.
3. Time is not sufficient to obtain consent from the subject's legal representative.
4. There is available no alternative method of approved or generally recognized therapy that provides an equal or greater likelihood of saving the life of the subject.

b. If immediate use of the test article is, in the investigator's opinion, required to preserve the life of the subject, and time is not sufficient to obtain the independent determination required in paragraph (a) of this section in advance of using the test article, the determinations of the clinical investigator shall be made and, within 5 working days after the use of the article, be reviewed and evaluated in writing by a physician who is not participating in the clinical investigation.

c. The documentation required in paragraph (a) or (b) of this section shall be submitted to the IRB within 5 working days after the use of the test article.

d. 1. The Commissioner may also determine that obtaining informed consent is not feasible when the Assistant Secretary of Defense (Health Affairs) requests such a determination in connection with the use of an investigational drug (including an antibiotic or biological product) in a specific protocol under an investigational new drug application (IND) sponsored by the Department of Defense (DOD). DOD's request for a determination that obtaining informed consent from military personnel is not feasible must be limited to a specific military operation involving combat or the immediate threat of combat. The request must also include a written justification supporting the conclusions of the physician(s) responsible for the medical care of the military personnel involved and the investigator(s) identified in the IND that a military combat exigency exists because of special military combat (actual or threatened) circumstances in which, in order to facilitate the accomplishment of the military mission, preservation of the health of the individual and the safety of other personnel require that a particular treatment be provided to a specified group of military personnel, without regard to what might be any individual's personal preference for no treatment or for some alternative treatment. The written request must also include a statement that a duly constituted institutional review board has reviewed and approved the use of the investigational drug without informed consent. The Commissioner may find that informed consent is not feasible only when withholding treatment would be contrary to the best interests of military personnel and there is no available satisfactory alternative therapy.

2. In reaching a determination under paragraph (d)(1) of this section that obtaining informed consent is not feasible and withholding treatment would be contrary to the best interests of military personnel, the Commissioner will review the request submitted under paragraph (d)(1) of this section and take into account all pertinent factors, including, but not limited to:

    i. The extent and strength of the evidence of the safety and effectiveness of the investigational drug for the intended use;

    ii. The context in which the drug will be administered, e.g., whether it is intended for use in a battlefield or hospital setting or whether it will be self-administered or will be administered by a health professional;

    iii. The nature of the disease or condition for which the preventive or therapeutic treatment is intended; and

    iv. The nature of the information to be provided to the recipients of the drug concerning the potential benefits and risks of taking or not taking the drug.

3. The Commissioner may request a recommendation from appropriate experts before reaching a determination on a request submitted under paragraph (d)(1) of this section.

4. A determination by the Commissioner that obtaining informed consent is not feasible and withholding treatment would be contrary to the best interests of military personnel will expire at the end of 1 year, unless renewed at DOD's request, or when DOD informs the Commissioner that the specific military operation creating the need for the use of the investigational drug has ended, whichever is earlier. The Commissioner may also revoke this determination based on changed circumstances.

[46 FR 8951, Jan. 27, 1981, as amended at 55 FR 52817, Dec. 21, 1990]

Sec. 50.24 Exception from informed consent requirements for emergency research.

a). The IRB responsible for the review, approval, and continuing review of the clinical investigation described in this section may approve that investigation without requiring that informed consent of all research subjects be obtained if the IRB (with the concurrence of a licensed physician who is a member of or consultant to the IRB and who is not otherwise participating in the clinical investigation) finds and documents each of the following:

1. The human subjects are in a life-threatening situation, available treatments are unproven or unsatisfactory, and the collection of valid scientific evidence, which may include evidence obtained

through randomized placebo-controlled investigations, is necessary to determine the safety and effectiveness of particular interventions.

2. Obtaining informed consent is not feasible because:
   i. The subjects will not be able to give their informed consent as a result of their medical condition;
   ii. The intervention under investigation must be administered before consent from the subjects' legally authorized representatives is feasible; and
   iii. There is no reasonable way to identify prospectively the individuals likely to become eligible for participation in the clinical investigation.

3. Participation in the research holds out the prospect of direct benefit to the subjects because:
   i. Subjects are facing a life-threatening situation that necessitates intervention;
   ii. Appropriate animal and other preclinical studies have been conducted, and the information derived from those studies and related evidence support the potential for the intervention to provide a direct benefit to the individual subjects; and
   iii. Risks associated with the investigation are reasonable in relation to what is known about the medical condition of the potential class of subjects, the risks and benefits of standard therapy, if any, and what is known about the risks and benefits of the proposed intervention or activity.

4. The clinical investigation could not practically be carried out without the waiver.

5. The proposed investigational plan defines the length of the potential therapeutic window based on scientific evidence, and the investigator has committed to attempting to contact a legally authorized representative for each subject within that window of time and, if feasible, to asking the legally authorized representative contacted for consent within that window rather than proceeding without consent. The investigator will summarize efforts made to contact legally authorized representatives and make this information available to the IRB at the time of continuing review.

6. The IRB has reviewed and approved informed consent procedures and an informed consent document consistent with Sec. 50.25. These procedures and the informed consent document are to be used with subjects or their legally authorized representatives in situations where use of such procedures and documents is feasible. The IRB has reviewed and approved procedures and information to be used when providing an opportunity for a family member to object to a subject's participation in the clinical investigation consistent with paragraph (a)(7)(v) of this section.

7. Additional protections of the rights and welfare of the subjects will be provided, including, at least:

    i.   Consultation (including, where appropriate, consultation carried out by the IRB) with representatives of the communities in which the clinical investigation will be conducted and from which the subjects will be drawn;

    ii.   Public disclosure to the communities in which the clinical investigation will be conducted and from which the subjects will be drawn, prior to initiation of the clinical investigation, of plans for the investigation and its risks and expected benefits;

    iii.   Public disclosure of sufficient information following completion of the clinical investigation to apprise the community and researchers of the study, including the demographic characteristics of the research population, and its results;

    iv.   Establishment of an independent data monitoring committee to exercise oversight of the clinical investigation; and

    v.   If obtaining informed consent is not feasible and a legally authorized representative is not reasonably available, the investigator has committed, if feasible, to attempting to contact within the therapeutic window the subject's family member who is not a legally authorized representative, and asking whether he or she objects to the subject's participation in the clinical investigation. The investigator will summarize efforts made to contact family members and make this information available to the IRB at the time of continuing review.

b.   The IRB is responsible for ensuring that procedures are in place to inform, at the earliest feasible opportunity, each subject, or if the subject remains incapacitated, a legally authorized representative of the subject, or if such a representative is not reasonably available, a family member, of the subject's inclusion in the clinical investigation, the details of the investigation and other information contained in the informed consent document. The IRB shall also ensure that there is a procedure to inform the subject, or if the subject remains incapacitated, a legally authorized representative of the subject, or if such a representative is not reasonably available, a family member, that he or she may discontinue the subject's participation at any time without penalty or loss of benefits to which the subject is otherwise entitled. If a legally authorized representative or family member is told about the clinical investigation and the subject's condition improves, the subject is also to be informed as soon as feasible. If a subject is entered into a clinical investigation with waived consent and the subject dies before a legally authorized representative or family member can be contacted, information about the clinical investigation is to be provided to the subject's legally authorized representative or family member, if feasible.

c.   The IRB determinations required by paragraph (a) of this section and the documentation required by paragraph (e) of this section are to be retained by the IRB for at least 3 years after completion of the clinical investigation, and the records shall be accessible for inspection and copying by FDA in accordance with Sec. 56.115(b) of this chapter.

d. Protocols involving an exception to the informed consent requirement under this section must be performed under a separate investigational new drug application (IND) or investigational device exemption (IDE) that clearly identifies such protocols as protocols that may include subjects who are unable to consent. The submission of those protocols in a separate IND/IDE is required even if an IND for the same drug product or an IDE for the same device already exists. Applications for investigations under this section may not be submitted as amendments under Secs. 312.30 or 812.35 of this chapter.

e. If an IRB determines that it cannot approve a clinical investigation because the investigation does not meet the criteria in the exception provided under paragraph (a) of this section or because of other relevant ethical concerns, the IRB must document its findings and provide these findings promptly in writing to the clinical investigator and to the sponsor of the clinical investigation. The sponsor of the clinical investigation must promptly disclose this information to FDA and to the sponsor's clinical investigators who are participating or are asked to participate in this or a substantially equivalent clinical investigation of the sponsor, and to other IRB's that have been, or are, asked to review this or a substantially equivalent investigation by that sponsor.

[61 FR 51528, Oct. 2, 1996]

Sec. 50.25 Elements of informed consent.

a. Basic elements of informed consent. In seeking informed consent, the following information shall be provided to each subject:

   1. A statement that the study involves research, an explanation of the purposes of the research and the expected duration of the subject's participation, a description of the procedures to be followed, and identification of any procedures which are experimental.

   2. A description of any reasonably foreseeable risks or discomforts to the subject.

   3. A description of any benefits to the subject or to others which may reasonably be expected from the research.

   4. A disclosure of appropriate alternative procedures or courses of treatment, if any, that might be advantageous to the subject.

   5. A statement describing the extent, if any, to which confidentiality of records identifying the subject will be maintained and that notes the possibility that the Food and Drug Administration may inspect the records.

   6. For research involving more than minimal risk, an explanation as to whether any compensation and an explanation as to whether any medical treatments are available if injury occurs and, if so, what they consist of, or where further information may be obtained.

7. An explanation of whom to contact for answers to pertinent questions about the research and research subjects' rights, and whom to contact in the event of a research-related injury to the subject.
8. A statement that participation is voluntary, that refusal to participate will involve no penalty or loss of benefits to which the subject is otherwise entitled, and that the subject may discontinue participation at any time without penalty or loss of benefits to which the subject is otherwise entitled.

b. Additional elements of informed consent. When appropriate, one or more of the following elements of information shall also be provided to each subject:

1. A statement that the particular treatment or procedure may involve risks to the subject (or to the embryo or fetus, if the subject is or may become pregnant) which are currently unforeseeable.
2. Anticipated circumstances under which the subject's participation may be terminated by the investigator without regard to the subject's consent.
3. Any additional costs to the subject that may result from participation in the research.
4. The consequences of a subject's decision to withdraw from the research and procedures for orderly termination of participation by the subject.
5. A statement that significant new findings developed during the course of the research which may relate to the subject's willingness to continue participation will be provided to the subject.
6. The approximate number of subjects involved in the study.

c. The informed consent requirements in these regulations are not intended to preempt any applicable Federal, State, or local laws which require additional information to be disclosed for informed consent to be legally effective.

d. Nothing in these regulations is intended to limit the authority of a physician to provide emergency medical care to the extent the physician is permitted to do so under applicable Federal, State, or local law.

Sec. 50.27 Documentation of informed consent.

a. Except as provided in Sec. 56.109(c), informed consent shall be documented by the use of a written consent form approved by the IRB and signed and dated by the subject or the subject's legally authorized representative at the time of consent. A copy shall be given to the person signing the form.

b. Except as provided in Sec. 56.109(c), the consent form may be either of the following:

1. A written consent document that embodies the elements of informed consent required by Sec. 50.25. This form may be read to the subject or the subject's legally authorized representative, but, in

any event, the investigator shall give either the subject or the representative adequate opportunity to read it before it is signed.

2. A short form written consent document stating that the elements of informed consent required by Sec. 50.25 have been presented orally to the subject or the subject's legally authorized representative. When this method is used, there shall be a witness to the oral presentation. Also, the IRB shall approve a written summary of what is to be said to the subject or the representative. Only the short form itself is to be signed by the subject or the representative. However, the witness shall sign both the short form and a copy of the summary, and the person actually obtaining the consent shall sign a copy of the summary. A copy of the summary shall be given to the subject or the representative in addition to a copy of the short form.

[46 FR 8951, Jan. 27, 1981, as amended at 61 FR 57280, Nov. 5, 1996]

Part 54

Financial Disclosure by Clinical Investigators

Authority: 21 U.S.C. 321, 331, 351, 352, 353, 355, 360, 360c-360j, 371, 372, 373, 374, 375, 376, 379; 42 U.S.C. 262.

Source: 63 FR 5250, Feb. 2, 1998, unless otherwise noted.

Sec. 54.1 Purpose.

a. The Food and Drug Administration (FDA) evaluates clinical studies submitted in marketing applications, required by law, for new human drugs and biological products and marketing applications and reclassification petitions for medical devices.

b. The agency reviews data generated in these clinical studies to determine whether the applications are approvable under the statutory requirements. FDA may consider clinical studies inadequate and the data inadequate if, among other things, appropriate steps have not been taken in the design, conduct, reporting, and analysis of the studies to minimize bias. One potential source of bias in clinical studies is a financial interest of the clinical investigator in the outcome of the study because of the way payment is arranged (e.g., a royalty) or because the investigator has a proprietary interest in the product (e.g., a patent) or because the investigator has an equity interest in the sponsor of the covered study. This section and conforming regulations require an applicant whose submission relies in part on clinical data to disclose certain financial arrangements between sponsor(s) of the covered studies and the clinical investigators and certain interests of the clinical investigators in the product under study or in the sponsor of the covered studies. FDA will use this information, in conjunction with information about the design and purpose of the study, as well as information obtained through on-site inspections, in the agency's assessment of the reliability of the data.

Sec. 54.2 Definitions.

For the purposes of this part:

a. Compensation affected by the outcome of clinical studies means compensation that could be higher for a favorable outcome than for an unfavorable outcome, such as compensation that is explicitly greater for a favorable result or compensation to the investigator in the form of an equity interest in the sponsor of a covered study or in the form of compensation tied to sales of the product, such as a royalty interest.

b. Significant equity interest in the sponsor of a covered study means any ownership interest, stock options, or other financial interest whose value cannot be readily determined through reference to public prices (generally, interests in a nonpublicly traded corporation), or any equity interest in a publicly traded corporation that exceeds $50,000 during the time the clinical investigator is carrying out the study and for 1 year following completion of the study.

c. Proprietary interest in the tested product means property or other financial interest in the product including, but not limited to, a patent, trademark, copyright or licensing agreement.

d. Clinical investigator means only a listed or identified investigator or subinvestigator who is directly involved in the treatment or evaluation of research subjects. The term also includes the spouse and each dependent child of the investigator.

e. Covered clinical study means any study of a drug or device in humans submitted in a marketing application or reclassification petition subject to this part that the applicant or FDA relies on to establish that the product is effective (including studies that show equivalence to an effective product) or any study in which a single investigator makes a significant contribution to the demonstration of safety. This would, in general, not include phase 1 tolerance studies or pharmacokinetic studies, most clinical pharmacology studies (unless they are critical to an efficacy determination), large open safety studies conducted at multiple sites, treatment protocols, and parallel track protocols. An applicant may consult with FDA as to which clinical studies constitute "covered clinical studies" for purposes of complying with financial disclosure requirements.

f. Significant payments of other sorts means payments made by the sponsor of a covered study to the investigator or the institution to support activities of the investigator that have a monetary value of more than $25,000, exclusive of the costs of conducting the clinical study or other clinical studies, (e.g., a grant to fund ongoing research, compensation in the form of equipment or retainers for ongoing consultation or honoraria) during the time the clinical investigator is carrying out the study and for 1 year following the completion of the study.

g. Applicant means the party who submits a marketing application to FDA for approval of a drug, device, or biologic product. The applicant is responsible for submitting the appropriate certification and disclosure statements required in this part.

h. Sponsor of the covered clinical study means the party supporting a particular study at the time it was carried out.

   [63 FR 5250, Feb. 2, 1998, as amended at 63 FR 72181, Dec. 31, 1998]

Sec. 54.3 Scope.

The requirements in this part apply to any applicant who submits a marketing application for a human drug, biological product, or device and who submits covered clinical studies. The applicant is responsible for making the appropriate certification or disclosure statement where the applicant either contracted with one or more clinical investigators to conduct the studies or submitted studies conducted by others not under contract to the applicant.

Sec. 54.4 Certification and disclosure requirements.

For purposes of this part, an applicant must submit a list of all clinical investigators who conducted covered clinical studies to determine whether the applicant's product meets FDA's marketing requirements, identifying those clinical investigators who are full-time or part-time employees of the sponsor of each covered study. The applicant must also completely and accurately disclose or certify information concerning the financial interests of a clinical investigator who is not a full-time or part-time employee of the sponsor for each covered clinical study. Clinical investigators subject to investigational new drug or investigational device exemption regulations must provide the sponsor of the study with sufficient accurate information needed to allow subsequent disclosure or certification. The applicant is required to submit for each clinical investigator who participates in a covered study, either a certification that none of the financial arrangements described in Sec. 54.2 exist, or disclose the nature of those arrangements to the agency. Where the applicant acts with due diligence to obtain the information required in this section but is unable to do so, the applicant shall certify that despite the applicant's due diligence in attempting to obtain the information, the applicant was unable to obtain the information and shall include the reason.

a. The applicant (of an application submitted under sections 505, 506, 510(k), 513, or 515 of the Federal Food, Drug, and Cosmetic Act, or section 351 of the Public Health Service Act) that relies in whole or in part on clinical studies shall submit, for each clinical investigator who participated in a covered clinical study, either a certification described in paragraph (a)(1) of this section or a disclosure statement described in paragraph (a)(3) of this section.

1. Certification: The applicant covered by this section shall submit for all clinical investigators (as defined in Sec. 54.2(d)), to whom the certification applies, a completed Form FDA 3454 attesting to the absence of financial interests and arrangements described in paragraph (a)(3) of this section. The form shall be dated and signed by the chief financial officer or other responsible corporate official or representative.

2. If the certification covers less than all covered clinical data in the application, the applicant shall include in the certification a list of the studies covered by this certification.

3. Disclosure Statement: For any clinical investigator defined in Sec. 54.2(d) for whom the applicant does not submit the certification described in paragraph (a)(1) of this section, the applicant shall submit a completed Form FDA 3455 disclosing completely and accurately the following:

    i. Any financial arrangement entered into between the sponsor of the covered study and the clinical investigator involved in the conduct of a covered clinical trial, whereby the value of the compensation to the clinical investigator for conducting the study could be influenced by the outcome of the study;

    ii. Any significant payments of other sorts from the sponsor of the covered study, such as a grant to fund ongoing research, compensation in the form of equipment, retainer for ongoing consultation, or honoraria;

    iii. Any proprietary interest in the tested product held by any clinical investigator involved in a study;

    iv. Any significant equity interest in the sponsor of the covered study held by any clinical investigator involved in any clinical study; and

    v. Any steps taken to minimize the potential for bias resulting from any of the disclosed arrangements, interests, or payments.

b. The clinical investigator shall provide to the sponsor of the covered study sufficient accurate financial information to allow the sponsor to submit complete and accurate certification or disclosure statements as required in paragraph (a) of this section. The investigator shall promptly update this information if any relevant changes occur in the course of the investigation or for 1 year following completion of the study.

c. Refusal to file application. FDA may refuse to file any marketing application described in paragraph (a) of this section that does not contain the information required by this section or a certification by the applicant that the applicant has acted with due diligence to obtain the information but was unable to do so and stating the reason.

[63 FR 5250, Feb. 2, 1998; 63 FR 35134, June 29, 1998, as amended at 64 FR 399, Jan. 5, 1999]

Sec. 54.5 Agency evaluation of financial interests.

a. Evaluation of disclosure statement. FDA will evaluate the information disclosed under Sec. 54.4(a)(2) about each covered clinical study in an application to determine the impact of any disclosed financial interests on the reliability of the study. FDA may consider both the size and nature of a disclosed financial interest (including the potential increase in the value of the interest if the product is approved) and steps that have been taken to minimize the potential for bias.

b. Effect of study design. In assessing the potential of an investigator's financial interests to bias a study, FDA will take into account the design and purpose of the study. Study designs that utilize such approaches as multiple investigators (most of whom do not have a disclosable interest), blinding, objective endpoints, or measurement of endpoints by someone other than the investigator may adequately protect against any bias created by a disclosable financial interest.

c. Agency actions to ensure reliability of data. If FDA determines that the financial interests of any clinical investigator raise a serious question about the integrity of the data, FDA will take any action it deems necessary to ensure the reliability of the data including:

 1. Initiating agency audits of the data derived from the clinical investigator in question;
 2. Requesting that the applicant submit further analyses of data, e.g., to evaluate the effect of the clinical investigator's data on overall study outcome;
 3. Requesting that the applicant conduct additional independent studies to confirm the results of the questioned study; and
 4. Refusing to treat the covered clinical study as providing data that can be the basis for an agency action.

Sec. 54.6 Recordkeeping and record retention.

a. Financial records of clinical investigators to be retained. An applicant who has submitted a marketing application containing covered clinical studies shall keep on file certain information pertaining to the financial interests of clinical investigators who conducted studies on which the application relies and who are not full or part-time employees of the applicant, as follows:

 1. Complete records showing any financial interest or arrangement as described in Sec. 54.4(a)(3)(i) paid to such clinical investigators by the sponsor of the covered study.
 2. Complete records showing significant payments of other sorts, as described in Sec. 54.4(a)(3)(ii), made by the sponsor of the covered clinical study to the clinical investigator.
 3. Complete records showing any financial interests held by clinical investigators as set forth in Sec. 54.4(a)(3)(iii) and (a)(3)(iv).

b. Requirements for maintenance of clinical investigators' financial records.

1. For any application submitted for a covered product, an applicant shall retain records as described in paragraph (a) of this section for 2 years after the date of approval of the application.
2. The person maintaining these records shall, upon request from any properly authorized officer or employee of FDA, at reasonable times, permit such officer or employee to have access to and copy and verify these records.

Part 56

Institutional Review Boards

Subpart A – General Provisions

Sec. 56.101 Scope.

a. This part contains the general standards for the composition, operation, and responsibility of an Institutional Review Board (IRB) that reviews clinical investigations regulated by the Food and Drug Administration under sections 505(i), 507(d), and 520(g) of the act, as well as clinical investigations that support applications for research or marketing permits for products regulated by the Food and Drug Administration, including food and color additives, drugs for human use, medical devices for human use, biological products for human use, and electronic products. Compliance with this part is intended to protect the rights and welfare of human subjects involved in such investigations.

b. References in this part to regulatory sections of the Code of Federal Regulations are to chapter I of title 21, unless otherwise noted.

Sec. 56.102 Definitions

As used in this part:

a. Act means the Federal Food, Drug, and Cosmetic Act, as amended (secs. 201-902, 52 Stat. 1040 et seq., as amended (21 U.S.C. 321-392)).

b. Application for research or marketing permit includes:
1. A color additive petition, described in part 71.
2. Data and information regarding a substance submitted as part of the procedures for establishing that a substance is generally recognized as safe for a use which results or may reasonably be expected to result, directly or indirectly, in its becoming a component or otherwise affecting the characteristics of any food, described in Sec. 170.35.
3. A food additive petition, described in part 171.

4. Data and information regarding a food additive submitted as part of the procedures regarding food additives permitted to be used on an interim basis pending additional study, described in Sec. 180.1.

5. Data and information regarding a substance submitted as part of the procedures for establishing a tolerance for unavoidable contaminants in food and food-packaging materials, described in section 406 of the act.

6. An investigational new drug application, described in part 312 of this chapter.

7. A new drug application, described in part 314.

8. Data and information regarding the bioavailability or bioequivalence of drugs for human use submitted as part of the procedures for issuing, amending, or repealing a bioequivalence requirement, described in part 320.

9. Data and information regarding an over-the-counter drug for human use submitted as part of the procedures for classifying such drugs as generally recognized as safe and effective and not misbranded, described in part 330.

10. Data and information regarding an antibiotic drug submitted as part of the procedures for issuing, amending, or repealing regulations for such drugs, described in Sec. 314.300 of this chapter.

11. An application for a biological product license, described in part 601.

12. Data and information regarding a biological product submitted as part of the procedures for determining that licensed biological products are safe and effective and not misbranded, as described in part 601.

13. An Application for an Investigational Device Exemption, described in parts 812 and 813.

14. Data and information regarding a medical device for human use submitted as part of the procedures for classifying such devices, described in part 860.

15. Data and information regarding a medical device for human use submitted as part of the procedures for establishing, amending, or repealing a standard for such device, described in part 861.

16. An application for premarket approval of a medical device for human use, described in section 515 of the act.

17. A product development protocol for a medical device for human use, described in section 515 of the act.

18. Data and information regarding an electronic product submitted as part of the procedures for establishing, amending, or repealing a standard for such products, described in section 358 of the Public Health Service Act.

19. Data and information regarding an electronic product submitted as part of the procedures for obtaining a variance from any electronic product performance standard, as described in Sec. 1010.4.

20. Data and information regarding an electronic product submitted as part of the procedures for granting, amending, or extending an exemption from a radiation safety performance standard, as described in Sec. 1010.5.
21. Data and information regarding an electronic product submitted as part of the procedures for obtaining an exemption from notification of a radiation safety defect or failure of compliance with a radiation safety performance standard, described in subpart D of part 1003.

c. Clinical investigation means any experiment that involves a test article and one or more human subjects, and that either must meet the requirements for prior submission to the Food and Drug Administration under section 505(i), 507(d), or 520(g) of the act, or need not meet the requirements for prior submission to the Food and Drug Administration under these sections of the act, but the results of which are intended to be later submitted to, or held for inspection by, the Food and Drug Administration as part of an application for a research or marketing permit. The term does not include experiments that must meet the provisions of part 58, regarding nonclinical laboratory studies. The terms research, clinical research, clinical study, study, and clinical investigation are deemed to be synonymous for purposes of this part.

d. Emergency use means the use of a test article on a human subject in a life-threatening situation in which no standard acceptable treatment is available, and in which there is not sufficient time to obtain IRB approval.

e. Human subject means an individual who is or becomes a participant in research, either as a recipient of the test article or as a control. A subject may be either a healthy individual or a patient.

f. Institution means any public or private entity or agency (including Federal, State, and other agencies). The term facility as used in section 520(g) of the act is deemed to be synonymous with the term institution for purposes of this part.

g. Institutional Review Board (IRB) means any board, committee, or other group formally designated by an institution to review, to approve the initiation of, and to conduct periodic review of, biomedical research involving human subjects. The primary purpose of such review is to assure the protection of the rights and welfare of the human subjects. The term has the same meaning as the phrase institutional review committee as used in section 520(g) of the act.

h. Investigator means an individual who actually conducts a clinical investigation (i.e., under whose immediate direction the test article is administered or dispensed to, or used involving, a subject) or, in the event of an investigation conducted by a team of individuals, is the responsible leader of that team.

i. Minimal risk means that the probability and magnitude of harm or discomfort anticipated in the research are not greater in and of themselves than those ordinarily encountered in daily life or during the performance of routine physical or psychological examinations or tests.

j. Sponsor means a person or other entity that initiates a clinical investigation, but that does not actually conduct the investigation, i.e., the test article is administered or dispensed to, or used involving, a subject under the immediate direction of another individual. A person other than an individual (e.g., a corporation or agency) that uses one or more of its own employees to conduct an investigation that it has initiated is considered to be a sponsor (not a sponsor-investigator), and the employees are considered to be investigators.

k. Sponsor-investigator means an individual who both initiates and actually conducts, alone or with others, a clinical investigation, i.e., under whose immediate direction the test article is administered or dispensed to, or used involving, a subject. The term does not include any person other than an individual, e.g., it does not include a corporation or agency. The obligations of a sponsor-investigator under this part include both those of a sponsor and those of an investigator.

l. Test article means any drug for human use, biological product for human use, medical device for human use, human food additive, color additive, electronic product, or any other article subject to regulation under the act or under sections 351 or 354-360F of the Public Health Service Act.

m. IRB approval means the determination of the IRB that the clinical investigation has been reviewed and may be conducted at an institution within the constraints set forth by the IRB and by other institutional and Federal requirements.
    [46 FR 8975, Jan. 27, 1981, as amended at 54 FR 9038, Mar. 3, 1989; 56 FR 28028, June 18, 1991]

Sec. 56.103 Circumstances in which IRB review is required.

a. Except as provided in Secs. 56.104 and 56.105, any clinical investigation which must meet the requirements for prior submission (as required in parts 312, 812, and 813) to the Food and Drug Administration shall not be initiated unless that investigation has been reviewed and approved by, and remains subject to continuing review by, anIRB meeting the requirements of this part.

b. Except as provided in Secs. 56.104 and 56.105, the Food and Drug Administration may decide not to consider in support of an application for a research or marketing permit any data or information that has been derived from a clinical investigation that has not been approved by, and that was not subject to initial and continuing review by, an IRB meeting the requirements of this part. The determination that a clinical investigation may not be considered in support of an application for a research or marketing permit does not, however, relieve the applicant for such a permit of any obligation under any other applicable regulations to submit the results of the investigation to the Food and Drug Administration.

c. Compliance with these regulations will in no way render inapplicable pertinent Federal, State, or local laws or regulations.
[46 FR 8975, Jan. 27, 1981; 46 FR 14340, Feb. 27, 1981]

Sec. 56.104 Exemptions from IRB requirement.

The following categories of clinical investigations are exempt from the requirements of this part for IRB review:

a. Any investigation which commenced before July 27, 1981 and was subject to requirements for IRB review under FDA regulations before that date, provided that the investigation remains subject to review of an IRB which meets the FDA requirements in effect before July 27, 1981.
b. Any investigation commenced before July 27, 1981 and was not otherwise subject to requirements for IRB review under Food and Drug Administration regulations before that date.
c. Emergency use of a test article, provided that such emergency use is reported to the IRB within 5 working days. Any subsequent use of the test article at the institution is subject to IRB review.
d. Taste and food quality evaluations and consumer acceptance studies, if wholesome foods without additives are consumed or if a food is consumed that contains a food ingredient at or below the level and for a use found to be safe, or agricultural, chemical, or environmental contaminant at or below the level found to be safe, by the Food and Drug Administration or approved by the Environmental Protection Agency or the Food Safety and Inspection Service of the U.S. Department of Agriculture.
[46 FR 8975, Jan. 27, 1981, as amended at 56 FR 28028, June 18, 1991]

Sec. 56.105 Waiver of IRB requirement.

On the application of a sponsor or sponsor-investigator, the Food and Drug Administration may waive any of the requirements contained in these regulations, including the requirements for IRB review, for specific research activities or for classes of research activities, otherwise covered by these regulations.

Subpart B – Organization and Personnel

Sec. 56.107 IRB membership.

a. Each IRB shall have at least five members, with varying backgrounds to promote complete and adequate review of research activities commonly conducted by the institution. The IRB shall be sufficiently qualified through the experience and expertise of its members, and the diversity of the members, including consideration of race, gender, cultural back-

grounds, and sensitivity to such issues as community attitudes, to promote respect for its advice and counsel in safeguarding the rights and
welfare of human subjects. In addition to possessing the professional
competence necessary to review the specific research activities, the IRB
shall be able to ascertain the acceptability of proposed research in terms
of institutional commitments and regulations, applicable law, and standards or professional conduct and practice. The IRB shall therefore
include persons knowledgeable in these areas. If an IRB regularly reviews
research that involves a vulnerable catgory of subjects, such as children,
prisoners, pregnant women, or handicapped or mentally disabled persons, consideration shall be given to the inclusion of one or more individuals who are knowledgeable about and experienced in working with
those subjects.

b. Every nondiscriminatory effort will be made to ensure that no IRB con-
sists entirely of men or entirely of women, including the instituton's consideration of qualified persons of both sexes, so long as no selection is
made to the IRB on the basis of gender. No IRB may consist entirely of
members of one profession.

c. Each IRB shall include at least one member whose primary concerns are
in the scientific area and at least one member whose primary concerns
are in nonscientific areas.

d. Each IRB shall include at least one member who is not otherwise affiliated with the institution and who is not part of the immediate family of a
person who is affiliated with the institution.

e. No IRB may have a member participate in the IRB's initial or continuing review of any project in which the member has a conflicting interest,
except to provide information requested by the IRB.

f. An IRB may, in its discretion, invite individuals with competence in special areas to assist in the review of complex issues which require expertise beyond or in addition to that available on the IRB. These individuals
may not vote with the IRB.

[46 FR 8975, Jan 27, 1981, as amended at 56 FR 28028, June 18, 1991; 56
FR 29756, June 28, 1991]

Subpart C – IRB Functions and Operations

Sec. 56.108 IRB functions and operations.

In order to fulfill the requirements of these regulations, each IRB shall:

a. Follow written procedures:

    1. For conducting its initial and continuing review of research and for
        reporting its findings and actions to the investigator and the institu-
        tion;

    2. for determining which projects require review more often than
        annually and which projects need verification from sources other

than the investigator that no material changes have occurred since previous IRB review;

3. for ensuring prompt reporting to the IRB of changes in research activity; and

4. for ensuring that changes in approved research, during the period for which IRB approval has already been given, may not be initiated without IRB review and approval except where necessary to eliminate apparent immediate hazards to the human subjects.

b. Follow written procedures for ensuring prompt reporting to the IRB, appropriate institutional officials, and the Food and Drug Administration of:

1. Any unanticipated problems involving risks to human subjects or others;

2. any instance of serious or continuing noncompliance with these regulations or the requirements or determinations of the IRB; or

3. any suspension or termination of IRB approval.

c. Except when an expedited review procedure is used (see Sec. 56.110), review proposed research at convened meetings at which a majority of the members of the IRB are present, including at least one member whose primary concerns are in nonscientific areas. In order for the research to be approved, it shall receive the approval of a majority of those members present at the meeting.

(Information collection requirements in this section were approved by the Office of Management and Budget (OMB) and assigned OMB control number 0910-0130)

[46 FR 8975, Jan. 27, 1981, as amended at 56 FR 28028, June 18, 1991]

Sec. 56.109 IRB review of research.

a. An IRB shall review and have authority to approve, require modifications in (to secure approval), or disapprove all research activities covered by these regulations.

b. An IRB shall require that information given to subjects as part of informed consent is in accordance with Sec. 50.25. The IRB may require that information, in addition to that specifically mentioned in Sec. 50.25, be given to the subjects when in the IRB's judgment the information would meaningfully add to the protection of the rights and welfare of subjects.

c. An IRB shall require documentation of informed consent in accordance with Sec. 50.27 of this chapter, except as follows:

1. The IRB may, for some or all subjects, waive the requirement that the subject, or the subject's legally authorized representative, sign a written consent form if it finds that the research presents no more than minimal risk of harm to subjects and involves no procedures for which written consent is normally required outside the research context; or

2. The IRB may, for some or all subjects, find that the requirements in Sec. 50.24 of this chapter for an exception from informed consent for emergency research are met.

d. In cases where the documentation requirement is waived under paragraph (c)(1) of this section, the IRB may require the investigator to provide subjects with a written statement regarding the research.

e. An IRB shall notify investigators and the institution in writing of its decision to approve or disapprove the proposed research activity, or of modifications required to secure IRB approval of the research activity. If the IRB decides to disapprove a research activity, it shall include in its written notification a statement of the reasons for its decision and give the investigator an opportunity to respond in person or in writing. For investigations involving an exception to informed consent under Sec. 50.24 of this chapter, an IRB shall promptly notify in writing the investigator and the sponsor of the research when an IRB determines that it cannot approve the research because it does not meet the criteria in the exception provided under Sec. 50.24(a) of this chapter or because of other relevant ethical concerns. The written notification shall include a statement of the reasons for the IRB's determination.

f. An IRB shall conduct continuing review of research covered by these regulations at intervals appropriate to the degree of risk, but not less than once per year, and shall have authority to observe or have a third party observe the consent process and the research.

g. An IRB shall provide in writing to the sponsor of research involving an exception to informed consent under Sec. 50.24 of this chapter a copy of information that has been publicly disclosed under Sec. 50.24(a)(7)(ii) and (a)(7)(iii) of this chapter. The IRB shall provide this information to the sponsor promptly so that the sponsor is aware that such disclosure has occurred. Upon receipt, the sponsor shall provide copies of the information disclosed to FDA.

[46 FR 8975, Jan. 27, 1981, as amended at 61 FR 51529, Oct. 2, 1996]

Sec. 56.110 Expedited review procedures for certain kinds of research involving no more than minimal risk, and for minor changes in approved research.

a. The Food and Drug Administration has established, and published in the Federal Register, a list of categories of research that may be reviewed by the IRB through an expedited review procedure. The list will be amended, as appropriate, through periodic republication in the Federal Register.

b. An IRB may use the expedited review procedure to review either or both of the following:

1. Some or all of the research appearing on the list and found by the reviewer(s) to involve no more than minimal risk,

2. minor changes in previously approved research during the period (of 1 year or less) for which approval is authorized. Under an expe-

dited review procedure, the review may be carried out by the IRB chairperson or by one or more experienced reviewers designated by the IRB chairperson from among the members of the IRB. In reviewing the research, the reviewers may exercise all of the authorities of the IRB except that the reviewers may not disapprove the research. A research activity may be disapproved only after review in accordance with the nonexpedited review procedure set forth in Sec. 56.108(c).

c. Each IRB which uses an expedited review procedure shall adopt a method for keeping all members advised of research proposals which have been approved under the procedure.

d. The Food and Drug Administration may restrict, suspend, or terminate an institution's or IRB's use of the expedited review procedure when necessary to protect the rights or welfare of subjects.

[46 FR 8975, Jan. 27, 1981, as amended at 56 FR 28029, June 18, 1991]

Sec. 56.111 Criteria for IRB approval of research.

a. In order to approve research covered by these regulations the IRB shall determine that all of the following requirements are satisfied:
   1. Risks to subjects are minimized:
      i. By using procedures which are consistent with sound research design and which do not unnecessarily expose subjects to risk, and
      ii. whenever appropriate, by using procedures already being performed on the subjects for diagnostic or treatment purposes.
   2. Risks to subjects are reasonable in relation to anticipated benefits, if any, to subjects, and the importance of the knowledge that may be expected to result. In evaluating risks and benefits, the IRB should consider only those risks and benefits that may result from the research (as distinguished from risks and benefits of therapies that subjects would receive even if not participating in the research). The IRB should not consider possible long-range effects of applying knowledge gained in the research (for example, the possible effects of the research on public policy) as among those research risks that fall within the purview of its responsibility.
   3. Selection of subjects is equitable. In making this assessment the IRB should take into account the purposes of the research and the setting in which the research will be conducted and should be particularly cognizant of the special problems of research involving vulnerable populations, such as children, prisoners, pregnant women, handicapped, or mentally disabled persons, or economically or educationally disadvantaged persons.
   4. Informed consent will be sought from each prospective subject or the subject's legally authorized representative, in accordance with and to the extent required by part 50.

5. Informed consent will be appropriately documented, in accordance with and to the extent required by Sec. 50.27.
6. Where appropriate, the research plan makes adequate provision for monitoring the data collected to ensure the safety of subjects.
7. Where appropriate, there are adequate provisions to protect the privacy of subjects and to maintain the confidentiality of data.

b. When some or all of the subjects, such as children, prisoners, pregnant women, handicapped, or mentally disabled persons, or economically or educationally disadvantaged persons, are likely to be vulnerable to coercion or undue influence additional safeguards have been included in the study to protect the rights and welfare of these subjects.

[46 FR 8975, Jan. 27, 1981, as amended at 56 FR 28029, June 18, 1991]

Part 312

Investigational New Drug Application

Subpart A – General Provisions

Sec. 312.1 Scope.

a. This part contains procedures and requirements governing the use of investigational new drugs, including procedures and requirements for the submission to, and review by, the Food and Drug Administration of investigational new drug applications (IND's). An investigational new drug for which an IND is in effect in accordance with this part is exempt from the premarketing approval requirements that are otherwise applicable and may be shipped lawfully for the purpose of conducting clinical investigations of that drug.

b. References in this part to regulations in the Code of Federal Regulations are to chapter I of title 21, unless otherwise noted.

Sec. 312.2 Applicability.

a. Applicability. Except as provided in this section, this part applies to all clinical investigations of products that are subject to section 505 or 507 of the Federal Food, Drug, and Cosmetic Act or to the licensing provisions of the Public Health Service Act (58 Stat. 632, as amended (42 U.S.C. 201 et seq.)).

b. Exemptions.
1. The clinical investigation of a drug product that is lawfully marketed in the United States is exempt from the requirements of this part if all the following apply:

     i.   The investigation is not intended to be reported to FDA as a well-controlled study in support of a new indication for use nor intended to be used to support any other significant change in the labeling for the drug;

    ii.   If the drug that is undergoing investigation is lawfully marketed as a prescription drug product, the investigation is not intended to support a significant change in the advertising for the product;

    iii.   The investigation does not involve a route of administration or dosage level or use in a patient population or other factor that significantly increases the risks (or decreases the acceptability of the risks) associated with the use of the drug product;

    iv.   The investigation is conducted in compliance with the requirements for institutional review set forth in part 56 and with the requirements for informed consent set forth in part 50; and

    v.   The investigation is conducted in compliance with the requirements of Sec. 312.7.

2.   i.   A clinical investigation involving an in vitro diagnostic biological product listed in paragraph (b)(2)(ii) of this section is exempt from the requirements of this part if (a) it is intended to be used in a diagnostic procedure that confirms the diagnosis made by another, medically established, diagnostic product or procedure and (b) it is shipped in compliance with Sec. 312.160.

    ii.   In accordance with paragraph (b)(2)(i) of this section, the following products are exempt from the requirements of this part:

    A.   blood grouping serum;

    B.   reagent red blood cells; and

    C.   anti-human globulin.

3.   A drug intended solely for tests in vitro or in laboratory research animals is exempt from the requirements of this part if shipped in accordance with Sec. 312.160.

4.   FDA will not accept an application for an investigation that is exempt under the provisions of paragraph (b)(1) of this section.

5.   A clinical investigation involving use of a placebo is exempt from the requirements of this part if the investigation does not otherwise require submission of an IND.

6.   A clinical investigation involving an exception from informed consent under Sec. 50.24 of this chapter is not exempt from the requirements of this part.

c.   Bioavailability studies. The applicability of this part to in vivo bioavailability studies in humans is subject to the provisions of Sec. 320.31.

d.   Unlabeled indication. This part does not apply to the use in the practice of medicine for an unlabeled indication of a new drug or antibiotic drug product approved under part 314 or of a licensed biological product.

e.   Guidance. FDA may, on its own initiative, issue guidance on the applicability of this part to particular investigational uses of drugs. On request, FDA will advise on the applicability of this part to a planned clinical investigation.

[52 FR 8831, Mar. 19, 1987, as amended at 61 FR 51529, Oct. 2, 1996]

Sec. 312.3 Definitions and interpretations.

a. The definitions and interpretations of terms contained in section 201 of the Act apply to those terms when used in this part:

b. The following definitions of terms also apply to this part: Act means the Federal Food, Drug, and Cosmetic Act (secs. 201-902, 52 Stat. 1040 et seq., as amended (21 U.S.C. 301-392)).

- *Clinical investigation* means any experiment in which a drug is administered or dispensed to, or used involving, one or more human subjects. For the purposes of this part, an experiment is any use of a drug except for the use of a marketed drug in the course of medical practice.

- *Contract research organization* means a person that assumes, as an independent contractor with the sponsor, one or more of the obligations of a sponsor, e.g., design of a protocol, selection or monitoring of investigations, evaluation of reports, and preparation of materials to be submitted to the Food and Drug Administration.

- *FDA* means the Food and Drug Administration.

- *IND* means an investigational new drug application. For purposes of this part, "IND" is synonymous with "Notice of Claimed Investigational Exemption for a New Drug."

- *Investigational new drug* means a new drug, antibiotic drug, or biological drug that is used in a clinical investigation. The term also includes a biological product that is used in vitro for diagnostic purposes. The terms "investigational drug" and "investigational new drug" are deemed to be synonymous for purposes of this part.

- *Investigator* means an individual who actually conducts a clinical investigation (i.e., under whose immediate direction the drug is administered or dispensed to a subject). In the event an investigation is conducted by a team of individuals, the investigator is the responsible leader of the team. "Subinvestigator" includes any other individual member of that team.

- *Marketing application* means an application for a new drug submitted under section 505(b) of the Act, a request to provide for certification of an antibiotic submitted under section 507 of the Act, or a product license application for a biological product submitted under the Public Health Service Act.

- *Sponsor* means a person who takes responsibility for and initiates a clinical investigation. The sponsor may be an individual or pharmaceutical company, governmental agency, academic institution, private organization, or other organization. The sponsor does not actually conduct the investigation unless the sponsor is a sponsor-investigator. A person other than an individual that uses one or more of its own employees to conduct an investigation that it has initiated is a sponsor, not a sponsor-investigator, and the employees are investigators.

- *Sponsor-Investigator* means an individual who both initiates and conducts an investigation, and under whose immediate direction the investigational drug is administered or dispensed. The term does not include any person other than an individual. The requirements applicable to a sponsor-investigator under this part include both those applicable to an investigator and a sponsor.

- *Subject* means a human who participates in an investigation, either as a recipient of the investigational new drug or as a control. A subject may be a healthy human or a patient with a disease.

Sec. 312.6 Labeling of an investigational new drug.

a. The immediate package of an investigational new drug intended for human use shall bear a label with thestatement "Caution: New Drug – Limited by Federal (or United States) law to investigational use."

b. The label or labeling of an investigational new drug shall not bear any statement that is false or misleading in any particular and shall not represent that the investigational new drug is safe or effective for the purposes for which it is being investigated.

Sec. 312.7 Promotion and charging for investigational drugs.

a. Promotion of an investigational new drug. A sponsor or investigator, or any person acting on behalf of a sponsor or investigator, shall not represent in a promotional context that an investigational new drug is safe or effective for the purposes for which it is under investigation or otherwise promote the drug. This provision is not intended to restrict the full exchange of scientific information concerning the drug, including dissemination of scientific findings in scientific or lay media. Rather, its intent is to restrict promotional claims of safety or effectiveness of the drug for a use for which it is under investigation and to preclude commercialization of the drug before it is approved for commercial distribution.

b. Commercial distribution of an investigational new drug. A sponsor or investigator shall not commercially distribute or test market an investigational new drug.

c. Prolonging an investigation. A sponsor shall not unduly prolong an investigation after finding that the results of the investigation appear to establish sufficient data to support a marketing application.

d. Charging for and commercialization of investigational drugs –
   1. Clinical trials under an IND. Charging for an investigational drug in a clinical trial under an IND is not permitted without the prior written approval of FDA. In requesting such approval, the sponsor shall provide a full written explanation of why charging is necessary in order for the sponsor to undertake or continue the clinical trial, e.g.,

why distribution of the drug to test subjects should not be considered part of the normal cost of doing business.

2. Treatment protocol or treatment IND. A sponsor or investigator may charge for an investigational drug for a treatment use under a treatment protocol or treatment IND provided:

    i. There is adequate enrollment in the ongoing clinical investigations under the authorized IND;

    ii. charging does not constitute commercial marketing of a new drug for which a marketing application has not been approved;

    iii. the drug is not being commercially promoted or advertised; and

    iv. the sponsor of the drug is actively pursuing marketing approval with due diligence. FDA must be notified in writing in advance of commencing any such charges, in an information amendment submitted under Sec. 312.31. Authorization for charging goes into effect automatically 30 days after receipt by FDA of the information amendment, unless the sponsor is notified to the contrary.

3. Noncommercialization of investigational drug. Under this section, the sponsor may not commercialize an investigational drug by charging a price larger than that necessary to recover costs of manufacture, research, development, and handling of the investigational drug.

4. Withdrawal of authorization. Authorization to charge for an investigational drug under this section may be withdrawn by FDA if the agency finds that the conditions underlying the authorization are no longer satisfied.

(Collection of information requirements approved by the Office of Management and Budget under control number 0910-0014)

[52 FR 8831, Mar. 19, 1987, as amended at 52 FR 19476, May 22, 1987]

Sec. 312.10 Waivers.

a. A sponsor may request FDA to waive applicable requirement under this part. A waiver request may be submitted either in an IND or in an information amendment to an IND. In an emergency, a request may be made by telephone or other rapid communication means. A waiver request is required to contain at least one of the following:

    1. An explanation why the sponsor's compliance with the requirement is unnecessary or cannot be achieved;

    2. A description of an alternative submission or course of action that satisfies the purpose of the requirement; or

    3. Other information justifying a waiver.

b. FDA may grant a waiver if it finds that the sponsor's noncompliance would not pose a significant and unreasonable risk to human subjects of the investigation and that one of the following is met:

1. The sponsor's compliance with the requirement is unnecessary for the agency to evaluate the application, or compliance cannot be achieved;
2. The sponsor's proposed alternative satisfies the requirement; or
3. The applicant's submission otherwise justifies a waiver.

(Collection of information requirements approved by the Office of Management and Budget under control number 0910-0014)

[52 FR 8831, Mar. 19, 1987, as amended at 52 FR 23031, June 17, 1987]

Subpart B – Investigational New Drug Application (IND)

Sec. 312.20 Requirement for an IND.

a. A sponsor shall submit an IND to FDA if the sponsor intends to conduct a clinical investigation with an investigational new drug that is subject to Sec. 312.2(a).
b. A sponsor shall not begin a clinical investigation subject to Sec. 312.2(a) until the investigation is subject to an IND which is in effect in accordance with Sec. 312.40.
c. A sponsor shall submit a separate IND for any clinical investigation involving an exception from informed consent under Sec. 50.24 of this chapter. Such a clinical investigation is not permitted to proceed without the prior written authorization from FDA.

FDA shall provide a written determination 30 days after FDA receives the IND or earlier.

[52 FR 8831, Mar. 19, 1987, as amended at 61 FR 51529, Oct. 2, 1996; 62 FR 32479, June 16, 1997]

Sec. 312.21 Phases of an investigation.

An IND may be submitted for one or more phases of an investigation. The clinical investigation of a previously untested drug is generally divided into three phases. Although in general the phases are conducted sequentially, they may overlap. These three phases of an investigation are a follows:

a. Phase 1.
   1. Phase 1 includes the initial introduction of an investigational new drug into humans. Phase 1 studies are typically closely monitored and may be conducted in patients or normal volunteer subjects. These studies are designed to determine the metabolism and pharmacologic actions of the drug in humans, the side effects associated with increasing doses, and, if possible, to gain early evidence on effectiveness. During Phase 1, sufficient information about the drug's pharmacokinetics and pharmacological effects should be obtained to permit the design of well-controlled, scientifically valid, Phase 2 studies. The total number of subjects and patients included in Phase

1 studies varies with the drug, but is generally in the range of 20 to 80.

2. Phase 1 studies also include studies of drug metabolism, structure-activity relationships, and mechanism of action in humans, as well as studies in which investigational drugs are used as research tools to explore biological phenomena or disease processes.

b. Phase 2. Phase 2 includes the controlled clinical studies conducted to evaluate the effectiveness of the drug for a particular indication or indications in patients with the disease or condition under study and to determine the common short-term side effects and risks associated with the drug. Phase 2 studies are typically well controlled, closely monitored, and conducted in a relatively small number of patients, usually involving no more than several hundred subjects.

c. Phase 3. Phase 3 studies are expanded controlled and uncontrolled trials. They are performed after preliminary evidence suggesting effectiveness of the drug has been obtained, and are intended to gather the additional information about effectiveness and safety that is needed to evaluate the overall benefit-risk relationship of the drug and to provide an adequate basis for physician labeling. Phase 3 studies usually include from several hundred to several thousand subjects.

Sec. 312.22 General principles of the IND submission.

a. FDA's primary objectives in reviewing an IND are, in all phases of the investigation, to assure the safety and rights of subjects, and, in Phase 2 and 3, to help assure that the quality of the scientific evaluation of drugs is adequate to permit an evaluation of the drug's effectiveness and safety. Therefore, although FDA's review of Phase 1 submissions will focus on assessing the safety of Phase 1 investigations, FDA's review of Phases 2 and 3 submissions will also include an assessment of the scientific quality of the clinical investigations and the likelihood that the investigations will yield data capable of meeting statutory standards for marketing approval.

b. The amount of information on a particular drug that must be submitted in an IND to assure the accomplishment of the objectives described in paragraph (a) of this section depends upon such factors as the novelty of the drug, the extent to which it has been studied previously, the known or suspected risks, and the developmental phase of the drug.

c. The central focus of the initial IND submission should be on the general investigational plan and the protocols for specific human studies. Subsequent amendments to the IND that contain new or revised protocols should build logically on previous submissions and should be supported by additional information, including the results of animal toxicology studies or other human studies as appropriate. Annual reports to the IND should serve as the focus for reporting the status of studies being conducted under the IND and should update the general investigational plan for the coming year.

d. The IND format set forth in Sec. 312.23 should be followed routinely by sponsors in the interest of fostering an efficient review of applications. Sponsors are expected to exercise considerable discretion, however, regarding the content of information submitted in each section, depending upon the kind of drug being studied and the nature of the available information. Section 312.23 outlines the information needed for a commercially sponsored IND for a new molecular entity. A sponsor-investigator who uses, as a research tool, an investigational new drug that is already subject to a manufacturer's IND or marketing application should follow the same general format, but ordinarily may, if authorized by the manufacturer, refer to the manufacturer's IND or marketing application in providing the technical information supporting the proposed clinical investigation. A sponsor-investigator who uses an investigational drug not subject to a manufacturer's IND or marketing application is ordinarily required to submit all technical information supporting the IND, unless such information may be referenced from the scientific literature.

Sec. 312.23 IND content and format.

a. A sponsor who intends to conduct a clinical investigation subject to this part shall submit an "Investigational New Drug Application" (IND) including, in the following order:
   1. Cover sheet (Form FDA-1571). A cover sheet for the application containing the following:
      i. The name, address, and telephone number of the sponsor, the date of the application, and the name of the investigational new drug.
      ii. Identification of the phase or phases of the clinical investigation to be conducted.
      iii. A commitment not to begin clinical investigations until an IND covering the investigations is in effect.
      iv. A commitment that an Institutional Review Board (IRB) that complies with the requirements set forth in part 56 will be responsible for the initial and continuing review and approval of each of the studies in the proposed clinical investigation and that the investigator will report to the IRB proposed changes in the research activity in accordance with the requirements of part 56.
      v. A commitment to conduct the investigation in accordance with all other applicable regulatory requirements.
      vi. The name and title of the person responsible for monitoring the conduct and progress of the clinical investigations.
      vii. The name(s) and title(s) of the person(s) responsible under Sec. 312.32 forreview and evaluation of information relevant to the safety of the drug.
      viii.If a sponsor has transferred any obligations for the conduct of any clinical study to a contract research organization, a state-

    ment containing the name and address of the contract research organization, identification of the clinical study, and a listing of the obligations transferred. If all obligations governing the conduct of the study have been transferred, a general statement of this transfer – in lieu of a listing of the specific obligations transferred – may be submitted.

  ix. The signature of the sponsor or the sponsor's authorized representative. If the person signing the application does not reside or have a place of business within the United States, the IND is required to contain the name and address of, and be countersigned by, an attorney, agent, or other authorized official who resides or maintains a place of business within the United States.

2. A table of contents.
3. Introductory statement and general investigational plan.
  i. A brief introductory statement giving the name of the drug and all active ingredients, the drug's pharmacological class, the structural formula of the drug (if known), the formulation of the dosage form(s) to be used, the route of administration, and the broad objectives and planned duration of the proposed clinical investigation(s).
  ii. A brief summary of previous human experience with the drug, with reference to other IND's if pertinent, and to investigational or marketing experience in other countries that may be relevant to the safety of the proposed clinical investigation(s).
  iii. If the drug has been withdrawn from investigation or marketing in any country for any reason related to safety or effectiveness, identification of the country(ies) where the drug was withdrawn and the reasons for the withdrawal.
  iv. A brief description of the overall plan for investigating the drug product for the following year. The plan should include the following: (a) The rationale for the drug or the research study; (b) the indication(s) to be studied; (c) the general approach to be followed in evaluating the drug; (d) the kinds of clinical trials to be conducted in the first year following the submission (if plans are not developed for the entire year, the sponsor should so indicate); (e) the estimated number of patients to be given the drug in those studies; and (f) any risks of particular severity or seriousness anticipated on the basis of the toxicological data in animals or prior studies in humans with the drug or related drugs.
4. [Reserved]
5. Investigator's brochure. If required under Sec. 312.55, a copy of the investigator's brochure, containing the following information:
  i. A brief description of the drug substance and the formulation, including the structural formula, if known.
  ii. A summary of the pharmacological and toxicological effects of the drug in animals and, to the extent known, in humans.

iii. A summary of the pharmacokinetics and biological disposition of the drug in animals and, if known, in humans.

iv. A summary of information relating to safety and effectiveness in humans obtained from prior clinical studies. (Reprints of published articles on such studies may be appended when useful.)

v. A description of possible risks and side effects to be anticipated on the basis of prior experience with the drug under investigation or with related drugs, and of precautions or special monitoring to be done as part of the investigational use of the drug.

6. Protocols.

i. A protocol for each planned study. (Protocols for studies not submitted initially in the IND should be submitted in accordance with Sec. 312.30(a).) In general, protocols for Phase 1 studies may be less detailed and more flexible than protocols for Phase 2 and 3 studies. Phase 1 protocols should be directed primarily at providing an outline of the investigation – an estimate of the number of patients to be involved, a description of safety exclusions, and a description of the dosing plan including duration, dose, or method to be used in determining dose – and should specify in detail only those elements of the study that are critical to safety, such as necessarymonitoring of vital signs and blood chemistries. Modifications of the experimental design of Phase 1 studies that do not affect critical safety assessments are required to be reported to FDA only in the annual report.

ii. In Phases 2 and 3, detailed protocols describing all aspects of the study should be submitted. A protocol for a Phase 2 or 3 investigation should be designed in such a way that, if the sponsor anticipates that some deviation from the study design may become necessary as the investigation progresses, alternatives or contingencies to provide for such deviation are built into the protocols at the outset. For example, a protocol for a controlled short-term study might include a plan for an early crossover of nonresponders to an alternative therapy.

iii. A protocol is required to contain the following, with the specific elements and detail of the protocol reflecting the above distinctions depending on the phase of study:

a. A statement of the objectives and purpose of the study.

b. The name and address and a statement of the qualifications (curriculum vitae or other statement of qualifications) of each investigator, and the name of each subinvestigator (e.g., research fellow, resident) working under the supervision of the investigator; the name and address of the research facilities to be used; and the name and address of each reviewing Institutional Review Board.

c. The criteria for patient selection and for exclusion of patients and an estimate of the number of patients to be studied.

d. A description of the design of the study, including the kind of control group to be used, if any, and a description of methods to be used to minimize bias on the part of subjects, investigators, and analysts.

e. The method for determining the dose(s) to be administered, the planned maximum dosage, and the duration of individual patient exposure to the drug.

f. A description of the observations and measurements to be made to fulfill the objectives of the study.

g. A description of clinical procedures, laboratory tests, or other measures to be taken to monitor the effects of the drug in human subjects and to minimize risk.

7. Chemistry, manufacturing, and control information.

i. As appropriate for the particular investigations covered by the IND, a section describing the composition, manufacture, and control of the drug substance and the drug product. Although in each phase of the investigation sufficient information is required to be submitted to assure the proper identification, quality, purity, and strength of the investigational drug, the amount of information needed to make that assurance will vary with the phase of the investigation, the proposed duration of the investigation, the dosage form, and the amount of information otherwise available. FDA recognizes that modifications to the method of preparation of the new drug substance and dosage form and changes in the dosage form itself are likely as the investigation progresses. Therefore, the emphasis in an initial Phase 1 submission should generally be placed on the identification and control of the raw materials and the new drug substance. Final specifications for the drug substance and drug product are not expected until the end of the investigational process.

ii. It should be emphasized that the amount of information to be submitted depends upon the scope of the proposed clinical investigation. For example, although stability data are required in all phases of the IND to demonstrate that the new drug substance and drug product are within acceptable chemical and physical limits for the planned duration of the proposed clinical investigation, if very short-term tests are proposed, the supporting stability data can be correspondingly limited.

iii. As drug development proceeds and as the scale or production is changed from the pilot-scale production appropriate for the limited initial clinical investigations to the larger-scale production needed for expanded clinical trials, the sponsor should submit information amendments to supplement the initial information submitted on the chemistry, manufacturing, and control processes with information appropriate to the expanded scope of the investigation.

iv. Reflecting the distinctions described in this paragraph (a)(7), and based on the phase(s) to be studied, the submission is required to contain the following:

   a. Drug substance. A description of the drug substance, including its physical, chemical, or biological characteristics; the name and address of its manufacturer; the general method of preparation of the drug substance; the acceptable limits and analytical methods used to assure the identity, strength, quality, and purity of the drug substance; and information sufficient to support stability of the drug substance during the toxicological studies and the planned clinical studies. Reference to the current edition of the United States Pharmacopeia – National Formulary may satisfy relevant requirements in this paragraph.

   b. Drug product. A list of all components, which may include reasonable alternatives for inactive compounds, used in the manufacture of the investigational drug product, including both those components intended to appear in the drug product and those which may not appear but which are used in the manufacturing process, and, where applicable, the quantitative composition of the investigational drug product, including any reasonable variations that may be expected during the investigational stage; the name and address of the drug product manufacturer; a brief general description of the manufacturing and packaging procedure as appropriate for the product; the acceptable limits and analytical methods used to assure the identity, strength, quality, and purity of the drug product; and information sufficient to assure the product's stability during the planned clinical studies. Reference to the current edition of the United States Pharmacopeia – National Formulary may satisfy certain requirements in this paragraph.

   c. A brief general description of the composition, manufacture, and control of any placebo used in a controlled clinical trial.

   d. Labeling. A copy of all labels and labeling to be provided to each investigator.

   e. Environmental analysis requirements. A claim for categorical exclusion under Sec. 25.30 or 25.31 or an environmental assessment under Sec. 25.40.

8. Pharmacology and toxicology information. Adequate information about pharmacological and toxicological studies of the drug involving laboratory animals or in vitro, on the basis of which the sponsor has concluded that it is reasonably safe to conduct the proposed clinical investigations. The kind, duration, and scope of animal and other tests required varies with the duration and nature of the proposed clinical investigations. Guidelines are available from FDA that

describe ways in which these requirements may be met. Such information is required to include the identification and qualifications of the individuals who evaluated the results of such studies and concluded that it is reasonably safe to begin the proposed investigations and a statement of where the investigations were conducted and where the records are available for inspection. As drug development proceeds, the sponsor is required to submit informational amendments, as appropriate, with additional information pertinent to safety.

i.   Pharmacology and drug disposition. A section describing the pharmacological effects and mechanism(s) of action of the drug in animals, and information on the absorption, distribution, metabolism, and excretion of the drug, if known.

ii. Toxicology.

    a. An integrated summary of the toxicological effects of the drug in animals and in vitro. Depending on the nature of the drug and the phase of the investigation, the description is to include the results of acute, subacute, and chronic toxicity tests; tests of the drug's effects on reproduction and the developing fetus; any special toxicity test related to the drug's particular mode of administration or conditions of use (e.g., inhalation, dermal, or ocular toxicology); and any in vitro studies intended to evaluate drug toxicity.

    b. For each toxicology study that is intended primarily to support the safety of the proposed clinical investigation, a full tabulation of data suitable for detailed review.

iii. For each nonclinical laboratory study subject to the good laboratory practice regulations under part 58, astatement that the study was conducted in compliance with the good laboratory practice regulations in part 58, or, if the study was not conducted in compliance with those regulations, a brief statement of the reason for the noncompliance.

9. Previous human experience with the investigational drug. A summary of previous human experience known to the applicant, if any, with the investigational drug. The information is required to include the following:

i.   If the investigational drug has been investigated or marketed previously, either in the United States or other countries, detailed information about such experience that is relevant to the safety of the proposed investigation or to the investigation's rationale. If the durg has been the subject of controlled trials, detailed information on such trials that is relevant to an assessment of the drug's effectiveness for the proposed investigational use(s) should also be provided. Any published material that is relevant to the safety of the proposed investigation or to an assessment of the drug's effectiveness for its proposed investigational use

should be provided in full. Published material that is less directly relevant may be supplied by a bibliography.
  ii. If the drug is a combination of drugs previously investigated or
      marketed, the information required under paragraph (a)(9)(i)
      of this section should be provided for each active drug compo-
      nent. However, if any component in such combination is subject
      to an approved marketing application or is otherwise lawfully
      marketed in the United States, the sponsor is not required to
      submit published material concerning that active drug compo-
      nent unless such material relates directly to the proosed investi-
      gational use (including publications relevant to component-
      component interaction).
  iii. If the drug has been marketed outside the United States, a list of
      the countries in which the drug has been marketed and a list of
      the countries in which the drug has been withdrawn from mar-
      keting for reasons potentially related to safety or effectiveness.
10. Additional information. In certain applications, as described below,
    information on special topics may be needed. Such information
    shall be submitted in this section as follows:
    i.   Drug dependence and abuse potential. If the drug is a psy-
         chotropic substance or otherwise has abuse potential, a section
         describing relevant clinical studies and experience and studies in
         test animals.
    ii. Radioactive drugs. If the drug is a radioactive drug, sufficient
         data from animal or human studies to allow a reasonable calcu-
         lation of radiation-absorbed dose to the whole body and critical
         organs upon administration to a human subject. Phase 1 studies
         of radioactive drugs must include studies which will obtain
         sufficient data for dosimetry calculations.
    iii. Other information. A brief statement of any other information
         that would aid evaluation of the proposed clinical investigations
         with respect to their safety or their design and potential as con-
         trolled clinical trials to support marketing of the drug.
11. Relevant information. If requested by FDA, any other relevant infor-
    mation needed for review of the application.
b. Information previously submitted. The sponsor ordinarily is not
   required to resubmit information previously submitted, but may incorporate the information by reference. A reference to information submitted previously must identify the file by name, reference number, volume,
   and page number where the information can be found. A reference to
   information submitted to the agency by a person other than the sponsor
   is required to contain a written statement that authorizes he reference
   and that is signed by the person who submitted the information.
c. Material in a foreign language. The sponsor shall submit an accurate and
   complete English translation of each part of the IND that is not in

English. The sponsor shall also submit a copy of each original literature publication for which an English translation is submitted.

d. Number of copies. The sponsor shall submit an original and two copies of all submissions to the IND file, including the original submission and all amendments and reports.

e. Numbering of IND submissions. Each submission relating to an IND isrequired to be numbered serially using a single, three-digit serial number. The initial IND is required to be numbered 000; each subsequent submission (e.g., amendment, report, or correspondence) is required to be numbered chronologically in sequence.

f. Identification of exception from informed consent. If the investigation involves an exception from informed consent under Sec. 50.24 of this chapter, the sponsor shall prominently identify on the cover sheet that the investigation is subject to the requirements in Sec. 50.24 of this chapter.

(Collection of information requirements approved by the Office of Management and Budget under control number 0910-0014)

[52 FR 8831, Mar. 19, 1987, as amended at 52 FR 23031, June 17, 1987; 53 FR 1918, Jan. 25, 1988; 61 FR 51529, Oct. 2, 1996; 62 FR 40599, July 29, 1997]

Sec. 312.30 Protocol amendments.

Once an IND is in effect, a sponsor shall amend it as needed to ensure that the clinical investigations are conducted according to protocols included in the application. This section sets forth the provisions under which new protocols may be submitted and changes in previously submitted protocols may be made. Whenever a sponsor intends to conduct a clinical investigation with an exception from informed consent for emergency research as set forth in Sec. 50.24 of this chapter, the sponsor shall submit a separate IND for such investigation.

a. New protocol. Whenever a sponsor intends to conduct a study that is not covered by a protocol already contained in the IND, the sponsor shall submit to FDA a protocol amendment containing the protocol for the study. Such study may begin provided two conditions are met:

   1. The sponsor has submitted the protocol to FDA for its review; and
   2. the protocol has been approved by the Institutional Review Board (IRB) with responsibility for review and approval of the study in accordance with the requirements of part 56. The sponsor may comply with these two conditions in either order.

b. Changes in a protocol.

   1. A sponsor shall submit a protocol amendment describing any change in a Phase 1 protocol that significantly affects the safety of subjects or any change in a Phase 2 or 3 protocol that significantly affects the safety of subjects, the scope of the investigation, or the scientific quality of the study. Examples of changes requiring an amendment under this paragraph include:

    i. Any increase in drug dosage or duration of exposure of individual subjects to the drug beyond that in the current protocol, or any significant increase in the number of subjects under study.

    ii. Any significant change in the design of a protocol (such as the addition or dropping of a control group).

    iii. The addition of a new test or procedure that is intended to improve monitoring for, or reduce the risk of, a side effect or adverse event; or the dropping of a test intended to monitor safety.

2. i. A protocol change under paragraph (b)(1) of this section may be made provided two conditions are met:

    a. The sponsor has submitted the change to FDA for its review; and

    b. The change has been approved by the IRB with responsibility for review and approval of the study. The sponsor may comply with these two conditions in either order.

    ii. Notwithstanding paragraph (b)(2)(i) of this section, a protocol change intended to eliminate an apparent immediate hazard to subjects may be implemented immediately provided FDA is subsequently notified by protocol amendment and the reviewing IRB is notified in accordance with Sec. 56.104(c).

c. New investigator. A sponsor shall submit a protocol amendment when a new investigator is added to carry out a previously submitted protocol, except that a protocol amendment is not required when a licensed practitioner is added in the case of a treatment protocol under Sec. 312.34. Once the investigator is added to the study, the investigational drug may be shipped to the investigator and the investigator may begin participating in the study. The sponsor shall notify FDA of the new investigator within 30 days of the investigator being added.

d. Content and format. A protocol amendment is required to be prominently identified as such (i.e., "Protocol Amendment: New Protocol", "Protocol Amendment: Change in Protocol", or "Protocol Amendment: New Investigator"), and to contain the following:

1. i. In the case of a new protocol, a copy of the new protocol and a brief description of the most clinically significant differences between it and previous protocols.

    ii. In the case of a change in protocol, a brief description of the change and reference (date and number) to the submission that contained the protocol.

    iii. In the case of a new investigator, the investigator's name, the qualifications to conduct the investigation, reference to the previously submitted protocol, and all additional information about the investigator's study as is required under Sec. 312.23(a)(6)(iii)(b).

2. Reference, if necessary, to specific technical information in the IND or in a concurrently submitted information amendment to the IND

that the sponsor relies on to support any clinically significant change in the new or amended protocol. If the reference is made to supporting information already in the IND, the sponsor shall identify by name, reference number, volume, and page number the location of the information.

3. If the sponsor desires FDA to comment on the submission, a request for such comment and the specific questions FDA's response should address.

e. When submitted. A sponsor shall submit a protocol amendment for a new protocol or a change in protocol before its implementation. Protocol amendments to add a new investigator or to provide additional information about investigators may be grouped and submitted at 30-dayintervals. When several submissions of new protocols or protocol changes are anticipated during a short period, the sponsor is encouraged, to the extent feasible, to include these all in a single submission.

(Collection of information requirements approved by the Office of Management and Budget under control number 0910-0014)

[52 FR 8831, Mar. 19, 1987, as amended at 52 FR 23031, June 17, 1987; 53 FR 1918, Jan. 25, 1988; 61 FR 51530, Oct. 2, 1996]

Sec. 312.31 Information amendments.

a. Requirement for information amendment. A sponsor shall report in an information amendment essential information on the IND that is not within the scope of a protocol amendment, IND safety reports, or annual report. Examples of information requiring an information amendment include:

1. New toxicology, chemistry, or other technical information; or
2. A report regarding the discontinuance of a clinical investigation.

b. Content and format of an information amendment. An information amendment is required to bear prominent identification of its contents (e.g., "Information Amendment: Chemistry, Manufacturing, and Control", "Information Amendment: Pharmacology-Toxicology", "Information Amendment: Clinical"), and to contain the following:

1. A statement of the nature and purpose of the amendment.
2. An organized submission of the data in a format appropriate for scientific review.
3. If the sponsor desires FDA to comment on an information amendment, a request for such comment.

c. When submitted. Information amendments to the IND should be submitted as necessary but, to the extent feasible, not more than every 30 days.

(Collection of information requirements approved by the Office of Management and Budget under control number 0910-0014)

[52 FR 8831, Mar. 19, 1987, as amended at 52 FR 23031, June 17, 1987; 53 FR 1918, Jan. 25, 1988]

Sec. 312.32 IND safety reports.

a. Definitions. The following definitions of terms apply to this section:-
Associated with the use of the drug. There is a reasonable possibility that
the experience may have been caused by the drug.

- *Disability*: A substantial disruption of a person's ability to conduct
normal life functions.

- *Life-threatening adverse drug experience*: Any adverse drug experience that places the patient or subject, in the view of the investigator, at immediate risk of death from the reaction as it occurred, i.e.,
it does not include a reaction that, had it occurred in a more severe
form, might have caused death.

- *Serious adverse drug experience*: Any adverse drug experience occurring at any dose that results in any of the following outcomes:
Death, a life-threatening adverse drug experience, inpatient hospitalization or prolongation of existing hospitalization, a persistent or
significant disability/incapacity, or a congenital anomaly/birth
defect. Important medical events that may not result in death, be
life-threatening, or require hospitalization may be considered a
serious adverse drug experience when, based upon appropriate
medical judgment, they may jeopardize the patient or subject and
may require medical or surgical intervention to prevent one of the
outcomes listed in this definition. Examples of such medical events
include allergic bronchospasm requiring intensive treatment in an
emergency room or at home, blood dyscrasias or convulsions that
do not result in inpatient hospitalization, or the development of
drug dependency or drug abuse.

- *Unexpected adverse drug experience*: Any adverse drug experience,
the specificity or severity of which is not consistent with the current investigator brochure; or, if an investigator brochure is not
required or available, the specificity or severity of which is not consistent with the risk information described in the general investigational plan or elsewhere in the current application, as amended.
For example, under this definition, hepatic necrosis would be
unexpected (by virtue of greater severity) if the investigator
brochure only referred to elevated hepatic enzymes or hepatitis.
Similarly, cerebral thromboembolism and cerebral vasculitis would
be unexpected (by virtue of greater specificity) if the investigator
brochure only listed cerebral vascular accidents. "Unexpected," as
used in this definition, refers to an adverse drug experience that has
not been previously observed (e.g., included in the investigator
brochure) rather than from the perspective of such experience not
being anticipated from the pharmacological properties of the pharmaceutical product.

b. Review of safety information. The sponsor shall promptly review all
information relevant to the safety of the drug obtained or otherwise
received by the sponsor from any source, foreign or domestic, including

information derived from any clinical or epidemiological investigations, animal investigations, commercial marketing experience, reports in the scientific literature, and unpublished scientific papers, as well as reports from foreign regulatory authorities that have not already been previously reported to the agency by the sponsor.

c. IND safety reports.
   1. Written reports
       i. The sponsor shall notify FDA and all participating investigators in a written IND safety report of:
           A. Any adverse experience associated with the use of the drug that is both serious and unexpected; or
           B. Any finding from tests in laboratory animals that suggests a significant risk for human subjects including reports of mutagenicity, teratogenicity, or carcinogenicity. Each notification shall be made as soon as possible and in no event later than 15 calendar days after the sponsor's initial receipt of the information. Each written notification may be submitted on FDA Form 3500A or in a narrative format (foreign events may be submitted either on an FDA Form 3500A or, if preferred, on a CIOMS I form; reports from animal or epidemiological studies shall be submitted in a narrative format) and shall bear prominent identification of its contents, i.e., "IND Safety Report." Each written notification to FDA shall be transmitted to the FDA new drug review division in the Center for Drug Evaluation and Research or the product review division in the Center for Biologics Evaluation and Research that has responsibilityfor review of the IND. If FDA determines that additional data are needed, the agency may require further data to be submitted.
       ii. In each written IND safety report, the sponsor shall identify all safety reports previously filed with the IND concerning a similar adverse experience, and shall analyze the significance of the adverse experience in light of the previouos, similar reports.
   2. Telephone and facsimile transmission safety reports. The sponsor shall also notify FDA by telephone or by facsimile transmission of any unexpected fatal or life-threatening experience associated with the use of the drug as soon as possible but in no event later than 7 calendar days after the sponsor's initial receipt of the information. Each telephone call or facsimile transmission to FDA shall be transmitted to the FDA new drug review division in the Center for Drug Evaluation and Research or the product review division in the Center for Biologics Evaluation and Research that has responsibility for review of the IND.
   3. Reporting format or frequency. FDA may request a sponsor to submit IND safety reports in a format or at a frequency different than that required under this paragraph. The sponsor may also propose

and adopt a different reporting format or frequency if the change is agreed to in advance by the director of the new drug review division in the Center for Drug Evaluation and Research or the director of the products review division in the Center for Biologics Evaluation and Research which is responsible for review of the IND.

4. A sponsor of a clinical study of a marketed drug is not required to make a safety report for any adverse experience associated with use of the drug that is not from the clinical study itself.

d. Followup.

1. The sponsor shall promptly investigate all safety information received by it.

2. Followup information to a safety report shall be submitted as soon as the relevant information is available.

3. If the results of a sponsor's investigation show that an adverse drug experience not initially determined to be reportable under paragraph (c) of this section is so reportable, the sponsor shall report such experience in a written safety report as soon as possible, but in no event later than 15 calendar days after the determination is made.

4. Results of a sponsor's investigation of other safety information shall be submitted, as appropriate, in an information amendment or annual report.

e. Disclaimer. A safety report or other information submitted by a sponsor under this part (and any release by FDA of that report or information) does not necessarily reflect a conclusion by the sponsor or FDA that the report or information constitutes an admission that the drug caused or contributed to an adverse experience. A sponsor need not admit, and may deny, that the report or information submitted by the sponsor constitutes an admission that the drug caused or contributed to an adverse experience.

(Collection of information requirements approved by the Office of Management and Budget under control number 0910-0014)

[52 FR 8831, Mar. 19, 1987, as amended at 52 FR 23031, June 17, 1987, 55 FR 11579, Mar. 29, 1990; 62 FR 52250, Oct. 7, 1997]

Effective Date Note: At 62 FR 52250, Oct. 7, 1997, Sec. 312.32 was amended by revising paragraphs (a), (b), (c)(1)(i), (c)(2), and (d)(3); by adding in the second sentence of paragraph (c)(3) the words "new drug review" before the phrase "division in the Center for Drug Evaluation and Research" and the words "the director of the product review division in" before the phrase "the Center for Biologics Evaluation and Research"; and by removing in paragraph (e) the word "section" and replacing it with the word "part", effective Apr. 6, 1998. For the convenience of the user, the superseded text is set forth as follows:

Sec. 312.32 IND safety reports.

a. Definitions. The following definitions of terms apply to this section:

Associated with the use of the drug means that there is a reasonable possibility that the experience may have been caused by the drug.

- *Serious adverse experience* means any experience that suggests a significant hazard, contraindication, side effect, or precaution. With respect to human clinical experience, a serious adverse drug experience includes any experience that is fatal or life-threatening, is permanently disabling, requires inpatient hospitalization, or is a congenital anomaly, cancer, or overdose. With respect to results obtained from tests in laboratory animals, aserious adverse drug experience includes any experience suggesting a significant risk for human subjects, including any finding of mutagenicity, teratogenicity, or carcinogenicity.

- *Unexpected adverse experience* means any adverse experience that is not identified in nature, severity, or frequency in the current investigator brochure; or, if an investigator brochure is not required, that is not identified in nature, severity, or freuquency in the risk information described in the general investigational plan or elsewhere in the current application, as amended.

b. Review of safety information. The sponsor shall promptly review all information relevant to the safety of the drug obtained or otherwise received by the sponsor from any source, foreign or domestic, including information derived from clinical investigations, animal investigations, commercial marketing experience, reports in the scientific literature, and unpublished scientific papers.

c. IND safety reports.
1. Written reports.
    i. The sponsor shall notify FDA and all participating investigators in a written IND safety report of any adverse experience associated with use of the drug that is both serious and unexpected. Such notification shall be made as soon as possible and in no event later than 10 working days after the sponsor's initial receipt of the information. Each written notification shall bear prominent identification of its contents, i.e., "IND Safety Report." Each written notification to FDA shall be transmitted to the FDA division of the Center for Drug Evaluation and Research or the Center for Biologics Evaluation and Research which has responsibility for review of the IND.
    ii. * * *
2. Telephone report. The sponsor shall also notify FDA by telephone of any unexpected fatal or life-threatening experience associated with use of the drug in the clinical studies conducted under the IND no later than 3 working days after receipt of the information. Each telephone call to FDA shall be transmitted to the FDA division of the Center for Drug Evaluation and Research or the Center for Biologics Evaluation and Research which has responsibility for review of the IND. For purposes of this section, life-threatening means that the

patient was, in the view of the investigator, at immediate (emphasis added) risk of death from the reaction as it occurred, i.e., it does not include a reaction that, had it occurred in a more serious form, might have caused death. For example, drug-induced hepatitis that resolved without evidence of hepatic failure would not be considered life-threatening even though drug-induced hepatitis can be fatal.

d.   * * *

   3.   If the results of a sponsor's investigation show that an adverse experience not initially determined to be reportable under paragraph (c) of this section is so reportable, the sponsor shall report such experience in a safety report as soon as possible after the determination is made, but in no event longer than 10-working days.

Sec. 312.33 Annual reports.

A sponsor shall within 60 days of the anniversary date that the IND went into effect, submit a brief report of the progress of the investigation that includes:

a.   Individual study information. A brief summary of the status of each study in progress and each study completed during the previous year. The summary is required to include the following information for each study:

   1.   The title of the study (with any appropriate study identifiers such as protocol number), its purpose, a brief statement identifying the patient population, and a statement as to whether the study is completed.

   2.   The total number of subjects initially planned for inclusion in the study; the number entered into the study to date, tabulated by age group, gender, and race; the number whose participation in the study was completed as planned; and the number who dropped out of the study for any reason.

   3.   If the study has been completed, or if interim results are known, a brief description of any available study results.

b.   Summary information. Information obtained during the previous year's clinical and nonclinical investigations, including:

   1.   A narrative or tabular summary showing the most frequent and most serious adverse experiences by body system.

   2.   A summary of all IND safety reports submitted during the past year.

   3.   A list of subjects who died during participation in the investigation, with the cause of death for each subject.

   4.   A list of subjects who dropped out during the course of the investigation in association with any adverse experience, whether or not thought to be drug related.

   5.   A brief description of what, if anything, was obtained that is pertinent to an understanding of the drug's actions, including, for example, information about dose response, information from controlled trails, and information about bioavailability.

6. A list of the preclinical studies (including animal studies) completed or in progress during the past year and a summary of the major preclinical findings.

7. A summary of any significant manufacturing or microbiological changes made during the past year.

c. A description of the general investigational plan for the coming year to replace that submitted 1 year earlier. The general investigational plan shall contain the information required under Sec. 312.23(a)(3)(iv).

d. If the investigator brochure has been revised, a description of the revision and a copy of the new brochure.

e. A description of any significant Phase 1 protocol modifications made during the previous year and not previously reported to the IND ina protocol amendment.

f. A brief summary of significant foreign marketing developments with the drug during the past year, such as approval of marketing in any country or withdrawal or suspension from marketing in any country.

g. If desired by the sponsor, a log of any outstanding business with respect to the IND for which the sponsor requests or expects a reply, comment, or meeting.

(Collection of information requirements approved by the Office of Management and Budget under control number 0910-0014)

[52 FR 8831, Mar. 19, 1987, as amended at 52 FR 23031, June 17, 1987; 63 FR 6862, Feb. 11, 1998]

Effective Date Note: At 63 FR 6862, Feb. 11, 1998, Sec. 312.33 was amended by revising paragraph (a)(2), effective Aug. 10, 1998. For the convenience of the user, the superseded text is set forth as follows:

Sec. 312.33 Annual reports.

a. * * *

2. The total number of subjects initially planned for inclusion in the study, the number entered into the study to date, the number whose participation in the study was completed as planned, and the number who dropped out of the study for any reason.

Sec. 312.34 Treatment use of an investigational new drug.

a. General. A drug that is not approved for marketing may be underclinical investigation for a serious or immediately life-threatening disease condition in patients for whom no comparable or satisfactory alternative drug or other therapy is available. During the clinical investigation of the drug, it may be appropriate to use the drug in the treatment of patients not in the clinical trials, in accordance with a treatment protocol or treatment IND. The purpose of this section is to facilitate the availability of promising new drugs to desperately ill patients as early in the drug development process as possible, before general marketing begins, and to obtain additional data on the drug's safety and effectiveness. In the case of a serious disease, a drug ordinarily may be made available for treatment use under this section during Phase 3 investigations or after all clinical trials have been completed; however, in appropriate circumstances, a drug may be made available for treatment use during Phase 2. In the case of an immediately life-threatening disease, a drug may be made available for treatment use under this section earlier than Phase 3, but ordinarily not earlier than Phase 2. For purposes of this section, the "treatment use" of a drug includes the use of a drug for diagnostic purposes. If a protocol for an investigational drug meets the criteria of this section, the protocol is to be submitted as a treatment protocol under the provisions of this section.

b. Criteria.

1. FDA shall permit an investigational drug to be used for a treatment use under a treatment protocol or treatment IND if:

   i. The drug is intended to treat a serious or immediately life-threatening disease;

   ii. There is no comparable or satisfactory alternative drug or other therapy available to treat that stage of thedisease in the intended patient population;

   iii. The drug is under investigation in a controlled clinical trial under an IND in effect for the trial, or all clinical trials have been completed; and

   iv. The sponsor of the controlled clinical trial is actively pursuing marketing approval of the investigational drug with due diligence.

2. Serious disease. For a drug intended to treat a serious disease, the Commissioner may deny a request for treatment use under a treatment protocol or treatment IND if there is insufficient evidence of safety and effectiveness to support such use.

3. Immediately life-threatening disease.

   i. For a drug intended to treat an immediately life-threatening disease, the Commissioner may deny a request for treatment use of an investigational drug under a treatment protocol or treatment IND if the available scientific evidence, taken as a whole, fails to provide a reasonable basis for concluding that the drug:

      A. May be effective for its intended use in its intended patient population; or

      B. Would not expose the patients to whom the drug is to be administered to an unreasonable and significant additional risk of illness or injury.

   ii. For the purpose of this section, an "immediately life-threatening" disease means a stage of a disease in which there is a reasonable likelihood that death will occur within a matter of months or in which premature death is likely without early treatment.

c. Safeguards. Treatment use of an investigational drug is conditioned on the sponsor and investigators complying with the safeguards of the IND process, including the regulations governing informed consent (21 CFR part 50) and institutional review boards (21 CFR part 56) and the applicable provisions of part 312, including distribution of the drug through qualified experts, maintenance of adequate manufacturing facilities, and submission of IND safety reports.

d. Clinical hold. FDA may place on clinical hold a proposed or ongoing treatment protocol or treatment IND in accordance with Sec. 312.42.

[52 FR 19476, May 22, 1987, as amended at 57 FR 13248, Apr. 15, 1992]

Sec. 312.35 Submissions for treatment use.

a. Treatment protocol submitted by IND sponsor. Any sponsor of a clinical investigation of a drug who intends to sponsor a treatment use for the drug shall submit to FDA a treatment protocol under Sec. 312.34 if the sponsor believes the criteria of Sec. 312.34 are satisfied. If a protocol is not submitted under Sec. 312.34, but FDA believes that the protocol should have been submitted under this section, FDA may deem the protocol to be submitted under Sec. 312.34. A treatment use under a treatment protocol may begin 30 days after FDA receives the protocol or on earlier notification by FDA that the treatment use described in the protocol may begin.

   1. A treatment protocol is required to contain the following:
      i. The intended use of the drug.
      ii. An explanation of the rationale for use of the drug, including, as appropriate, either a list of what available regimens ordinarily should be tried before using the investigational drug or an explanation of why the use of the investigational drug is preferable to the use of available marketed treatments.
      iii. A brief description of the criteria for patient selection.
      iv. The method of administration of the drug and the dosages.
      v. A description of clinical procedures, laboratory tests, or other measures to monitor the effects of the drug and to minimize risk.

   2. A treatment protocol is to be supported by the following:
      i. Informational brochure for supplying to each treating physician.
      ii. The technical information that is relevant to safety and effectiveness of the drug for the intended treatment purpose. Information contained in the sponsor's IND may be incorporated by reference.
      iii. A commitment by the sponsor to assure compliance of all participating investigators with the informed consent requirements of 21 CFR part 50.

   3. A licensed practitioner who receives an investigational drug for treatment use under a treatment protocol is an "investigator" under the protocol and is responsible for meeting all applicable investigator responsibilities under this part and 21 CFR parts 50 and 56.

b. Treatment IND submitted by licensed practitioner.

1. If a licensed medical practitioner wants to obtain an investigational drug subject to a controlled clinical trial for a treatment use, the practitioner should first attempt to obtain the drug from the sponsor of the controlled trial under a treatment protocol. If the sponsor of the controlled clinical investigation of the drug will not establish a treatment protocol for the drug under paragraph (a) of this section, the licensed medical practitioner may seek to obtain the drug from the sponsor and submit a treatment IND to FDA requesting authorization to use the investigational drug for treatment use. A treatment use under a treatment IND may begin 30 days after FDA receives the IND or on earlier notification by FDA that the treatment use under the IND may begin. A treatment IND is required to contain the following:

   i. A cover sheet (Form FDA 1571) meeting Sec. 312.23(g)(1).
   ii. Information (when not provided by the sponsor) on the drug's chemistry, manufacturing, and controls, and prior clinical and nonclinical experience with the drug submitted in accordance with Sec. 312.23. A sponsor of a clinical investigation subject to an IND who supplies an investigational drug to a licensed medical practitioner for purposes of a separate treatment clinical investigation shall be deemed to authorize the incorporation-by-reference of the technical information contained in the sponsor's IND into the medical practitioner's treatment IND.
   iii. A statement of the steps taken by the practitioner to obtain the drug under a treatment protocol from the drug sponsor.
   iv. A treatment protocol containing the same information listed in paragraph (a)(1) of this section.
   v. A statement of the practitioner's qualifications to use the investigational drug for the intended treatment use.
   vi. The practitioner's statement of familiarity with information on the drug's safety and effectiveness derived from previous clinical and nonclinical experience with the drug.
   vii. Agreement to report to FDA safety information in accordance with Sec. 312.32.

2. A licensed practitioner who submits a treatment IND under this section is the sponsor-investigator for such IND and is responsible for meeting all applicable sponsor and investigator responsibilities under this part and 21 CFR parts 50 and 56.

   (Collection of information requirements approved by the Office of Management and Budget under control number 0910-0014)

   [52 FR 19477, May 22, 1987, as amended at 57 FR 13249, Apr. 15, 1992]

Sec. 312.36 Emergency use of an investigational new drug.

Need for an investigational drug may arise in an emergency situation that does not allow time for submission of an IND in accordance with Sec.

312.23 or Sec. 312.34. In such a case, FDA may authorize shipment of the drug for a specified use in advance of submission of an IND. A request for such authorization may be transmitted to FDA by telephone or other rapid communication means. For investigational biological drugs, the request should be directed to the Division of Biological Investigational New Drugs (HFB-230), Center for Biologics Evaluation and Research, 8800 Rockville Pike, Bethesda, MD 20892, (301) 443-4864. For all other investigational drugs, the request for authorization should be directed to the Document Management and Reporting Branch (HFD-53), Center for Drug Evaluation and Research, 5600 Fishers Lane, Rockville, MD 20857, (301) 443-4320. After normal working hours, eastern standard time, the request should be directed to the FDA Division of Emergency and Epidemiological Operations, (202) 857-8400. Except in extraordinary circumstances, such authorization will be conditioned on the sponsor making an appropriate IND submission as soonas practicable after receiving the authorization.
(Collection of information requirements approved by the Office of Management and Budget under control number 0910-0014)
[52 FR 8831, Mar. 19, 1987, as amended at 52 FR 23031, June 17, 1987; 55 FR 11579, Mar. 29, 1990]

Sec. 312.38 Withdrawal of an IND.
a. At any time a sponsor may withdraw an effective IND without prejudice.
b. If an IND is withdrawn, FDA shall be so notified, all clinical investigations conducted under the IND shall be ended, all current investigators notified, and all stocks of the drug returned to the sponsor or otherwise disposed of at the request of the sponsor in accordance with Sec. 312.59.
c. If an IND is withdrawn because of a safety reason, the sponsor shall promptly so inform FDA, all participating investigators, and all reviewing Institutional Review Boards, together with the reasons for such withdrawal.
    (Collection of information requirements approved by the Office of Management and Budget under control number 0910-0014)
    [52 FR 8831, Mar. 19, 1987, as amended at 52 FR 23031, June 17, 1987]

Subpart C – Administrative Actions

Sec. 312.40 General requirements for use of an investigational new drug in a clinical investigation.
a. An investigational new drug may be used in a clinical investigation if the following conditions are met:
    1. The sponsor of the investigation submits an IND for the drug to FDA; the IND is in effect under paragraph (b) of this section; and the sponsor complies with all applicable requirements in this part

    and parts 50 and 56 with respect to the conduct of the clinical investigations; and

  2. Each participating investigator conducts his or her investigation in compliance with the requirements of this part and parts 50 and 56.

b. An IND goes into effect:

  1. Thirty days after FDA receives the IND, unless FDA notifies the sponsor that the investigations described in the IND are subject to a clinical hold under Sec. 312.42; or

  2. On earlier notification by FDA that the clinical investigations in the IND may begin. FDA will notify the sponsor in writing of the date it receives the IND.

c. A sponsor may ship an investigational new drug to investigators named in the IND:

  1. Thirty days after FDA receives the IND; or

  2. On earlier FDA authorization to ship the drug.

d. An investigator may not administer an investigational new drug to human subjects until the IND goes into effect under paragraph (b) of this section.

Sec. 312.41 Comment and advice on an IND.

a. FDA may at any time during the course of the investigation communicate with the sponsor orally or in writing about deficiencies in the IND or about FDA's need for more data or information.

b. On the sponsor's request, FDA will provide advice on specific matters relating to an IND. Examples of such advice may include advice on the adequacy of technical data to support an investigational plan, on the design of a clinical trial, and on whether proposed investigations are likely to produce the data and information that is needed to meet requirements for a marketing application.

c. Unless the communication is accompanied by a clinical hold order under Sec. 312.42, FDA communications with a sponsor under this section are solely advisory and do not require any modification in the planned or ongoing clinical investigations or response to the agency. (Collection of information requirements approved by the Office of Management and Budget under control number 0910-0014) [52 FR 8831, Mar. 19, 1987, as amended at 52 FR 23031, June 17, 1987]

Sec. 312.42 Clinical holds and requests for modification.

a. General. A clinical hold is an order issued by FDA to the sponsor to delay a proposed clinical investigation or to suspend an ongoing investigation. The clinical hold order may apply to one or more of the investigations covered by an IND. When a proposed study is placed on clinical hold, subjects may not be given the investigational drug. When an ongoing study is placed on clinical hold, no new subjects may be recruited to the study and placed on the investigational drug; patients already in the study should be taken off therapy involving the investigational drug unless specifically permitted by FDA in the interest of patient safety.

b. Grounds for imposition of clinical hold –

   1. Clinical hold of a Phase 1 study under an IND. FDA may place a proposed or ongoing Phase 1 investigation on clinical hold if it finds that:

      i.   Human subjects are or would be exposed to an unreasonable and significant risk of illness or injury;

      ii. The clinical investigators named in the IND are not qualified by reason of their scientific training and experience to conduct the investigation described in the IND;

      iii. The investigator brochure is misleading, erroneous, or materially incomplete; or

      iv. The IND does not contain sufficient information required under Sec. 312.23 to assess the risks to subjects of the proposed studies.

   2. Clinical hold of a Phase 2 or 3 study under an IND. FDA may place a proposed or ongoing Phase 2 or 3 investigation on clinical hold if it finds that:

      i.   Any of the conditions in paragraph (b)(1)(i) through (iv) of this section apply; or

      ii. The plan or protocol for the investigation is clearly deficient in design to meet its stated objectives.

   3. Clinical hold of a treatment IND or treatment protocol.

      i.   Proposed use. FDA may place a proposed treatment IND or treatment protocol on clinical hold if it is determined that:

         A. The pertinent criteria in Sec. 312.34(b) for permitting the treatment use to begin are not satisfied; or

         B. The treatment protocol or treatment IND does not contain the information required under Sec. 312.35 (a) or (b) to make the specified determination under Sec. 312.34(b).

      ii. Ongoing use. FDA may place an ongoing treatment protocol or treatment IND on clinical hold if it is determined that:

         A. There becomes available a comparable or satisfactory alternative drug or other therapy to treat that stage of the disease in the intended patient population for which the investigational drug is being used;

         B. The investigational drug is not under investigation in a controlled clinical trial under an IND in effect for the trial and not all controlled clinical trials necessary to support a marketing application have been completed, or a clinical study under the IND has been placed on clinical hold:

         C. The sponsor of the controlled clinical trial is not pursuing marketing approval with due diligence;

         D. If the treatment IND or treatment protocol is intended for a serious disease, there is insufficient evidence of safety and effectiveness to support such use; or

E. If the treatment protocol or treatment IND was based on an immediately life-threatening disease, the available scientific evidence, taken as a whole, fails to provide a reasonable basis for concluding that the drug:

1. May be effective for its intended use in its intended population; or
2. Would not expose the patients to whom the drug is to be administered to an unreasonable and significant additional risk of illness or injury.

iii. FDA may place a proposed or ongoing treatment IND or treatment protocol on clinical hold if it finds that any of the conditions in paragraph (b)(4)(i) through (b)(4)(viii) of this section apply.

4. Clinical hold of any study that is not designed to be adequate and well-controlled. FDA may place a proposed or ongoing investigation that is not designed to be adequate and well-controlled on clinical hold if it finds that:

i. Any of the conditions in paragraph (b)(1) or (b)(2) of this section apply; or

ii. There is reasonable evidence the investigation that is not designed to be adequate and well-controlled is impeding enrollment in, or otherwise interfering with the conduct or completion of, a study that is designed to be anadequate and well-controlled investigation of the same or another investigational drug; or

iii. Insufficient quantities of the investigational drug exist to adequately conduct both the investigation that is not designed to be adequate and well-controlled and the investigations that are designed to be adequate and well controlled; or

iv. The drug has been studied in one or more adequate and well-controlled investigations that strongly suggest lack of effectiveness; or

v. Another drug under investigation or approved for the same indication and available to the same patient population has demonstrated a better potential benefit/risk balance; or

vi. The drug has received marketing approval for the same indication in the same patient population; or

vii. The sponsor of the study that is designed to be an adequate and well-controlled investigation is not actively pursuing marketing approval of the investigational drug with due diligence; or

viii. The Commissioner determines that it would not be in the public interest for the study to be conducted or continued. FDA ordinarily intends that clinical holds under paragraphs (b)(4)(ii), (b)(4)(iii) and (b)(4)(v) of this section would only apply to additional enrollment in nonconcurrently controlled trials rather than eliminating continued access to individuals already receiving the investigational drug.

5. Clinical hold of any investigation involving an exception from informed consent under Sec. 50.24 of this chapter. FDA may place a proposed or ongoing investigation involving an exception from informed consent under Sec. 50.24 of this chapter on clinical hold if it is determined that:

   i. Any of the conditions in paragraphs (b)(1) or (b)(2) of this section apply; or

   ii. The pertinent criteria in Sec. 50.24 of this chapter for such an investigation to begin or continue are not submitted or not satisfied.

c. Discussion of deficiency. Whenever FDA concludes that a deficiency exists in a clinical investigation that may be grounds for the imposition of clinical hold FDA will, unless patients are exposed to immediate and serious risk, attempt to discuss and satisfactorily resolve the matter with the sponsor before issuing the clinical hold order.

d. Imposition of clinical hold. The clinical hold order may be made by telephone or other means of rapid communication or in writing. The clinical hold order will identify the studies under the IND to which the hold applies, and will briefly explain the basis for the action. The clinical hold order will be made by or on behalf of the Division Director with responsibility for review of the IND. As soon as possible, and no more than 30 days after imposition of the clinical hold, the Division Director will provide the sponsor a written explanation of the basis for the hold.

e. Resumption of clinical investigations. If, by the terms of the clinical hold order, resumption of the affected investigation is permitted without prior notification by FDA once a stated correction or modification is made, the investigation may proceed as soon as the correction or modification is made. In all other cases, an investigation may only resume after the Division Director (or the Director's designee) with responsibility for review of the IND has notified the sponsor that the investigation may proceed. In these cases resumption of the affected investigation(s) will be authorized when the sponsor corrects the deficiency(ies) previously cited or otherwise satisfied the agency that the investigation(s) can proceed. Resumption of a study may be authorized by telephone or other means of rapid communication.

f. Appeal. If the sponsor disagrees with the reasons cited for the clinical hold, the sponsor may request reconsideration of the decision in accordance with Sec. 312.48.

g. Conversion of IND on clinical hold to inactive status. If all investigations covered by an IND remain on clinical hold for 1 year or more, the IND may be placed on inactive status by FDA under Sec. 312.45.

[52 FR 8831, Mar. 19, 1987, as amended at 52 FR 19477, May 22, 1987; 57 FR 13249, Apr. 15, 1992; 61 FR 51530, Oct. 2, 1996]

Sec. 312.44 Termination.

a. General. This section describes the procedures under which FDA may terminate an IND. If an IND is terminated, the sponsor shall end all clinical investigations conducted under the IND and recall or otherwise provide for the disposition of all unused supplies of the drug. A termination action may be based on deficiencies in the IND or in the conduct of an investigation under an IND. Except as provided in paragraph (d) of this section, a termination shall be preceded by a proposal to terminate by FDA and an opportunity for the sponsor to respond. FDA will, in general, only initiate an action under this section after first attempting to resolve differences informally or, when appropriate, through the clinical hold procedures described in Sec. 312.42.

b. Grounds for termination –

   1. Phase 1. FDA may propose to terminate an IND during Phase 1 if it finds that:

      i. Human subjects would be exposed to an unreasonable and significant risk of illness or unjury.

      ii. The IND does not contain sufficient information required under Sec. 312.23 to assess the safety to subjects of the clinical investigations.

      iii. The methods, facilities, and controls used for the manufacturing, processing, and packing of the investigational drug are inadequate to establish and maintain appropriate standards of identity, strength, quality, and purity as needed for subject safety.

      iv. The clinical investigations are being conducted in a manner substantially different than that described in the protocols submitted in the IND.

      v. The drug is being promoted or distributed for commercial purposes not justified by the requirements of the investigation or permitted by Sec. 312.7.

      vi. The IND, or any amendment or report to the IND, contains an untrue statement of a material fact or omits material information required by this part.

      vii. The sponsor fails promptly to investigate and inform the Food and Drug Administration and all investigators of serious and unexpected adverse experiences in accordance with Sec. 312.32 or fails to make any other report required under this part.

      viii. The sponsor fails to submit an accurate annual report of the investigations in accordance with Sec. 312.33.

      ix. The sponsor fails to comply with any other applicable requirement of this part, part 50, or part 56.

      x. The IND has remained on inactive status for 5 years or more.

      xi. The sponsor fails to delay a proposed investigation under the IND or to suspend an ongoing investigation that has been placed on clinical hold under Sec. 312.42(b)(4).

2. Phase 2 or 3. FDA may propose to terminate an IND during Phase 2 or Phase 3 if FDA finds that:
   i. Any of the conditions in paragraphs (b)(1)(i) through (b)(1)(xi) of this section apply; or
   ii. The investigational plan or protocol(s) is not reasonable as a bona fide scientific plan to determine whether or not the drug is safe and effective for use; or
   iii. There is convincing evidence that the drug is not effective for the purpose for which it is being investigated.
3. FDA may propose to terminate a treatment IND if it finds that:
   i. Any of the conditions in paragraphs (b)(1)(i) through (x) of this section apply; or
   ii. Any of the conditions in Sec. 312.42(b)(3) apply.

c. Opportunity for sponsor response.
   1. If FDA proposes to terminate an IND, FDA will notify the sponsor in writing, and invite correction or explanation within a period of 30 days.
   2. On such notification, the sponsor may provide a written explanation or correction or may request a conference with FDA to provide the requested explanation or correction. If the sponsor does not respond to the notification within the allocated time, the IND shall be terminated.
   3. If the sponsor responds but FDA does not accept the explanation or correction submitted, FDA shall inform the sponsor in writing of the reason for the nonacceptance and provide the sponsor with an opportunity for a regulatory hearing before FDA under part 16 on the question of whether the IND should be terminated. The sponsor's request for a regulatory hearing must be made within 10 days of the sponsor'sreceipt of FDA's notification of nonacceptance.

d. Immediate termination of IND. Notwithstanding paragraphs (a) through (c) of this section, if at any time FDA concludes that continuation of the investigation presents an immediate and substantial danger to the health of individuals, the agency shall immediately, by written notice to the sponsor from the Director of the Center for Drug Evaluation and Research or the Director of the Center for Biologics Evaluation and Research, terminate the IND. An IND so terminated is subject to reinstatement by the Director on the basis of additional submissions that eliminate such danger. If an IND is terminated under this paragraph, the agency will afford the sponsor an opportunity for a regulatory hearing under part 16 on the question of whether the IND should be reinstated.

(Collection of information requirements approved by the Office of Management and Budget under control number 0910-0014)

[52 FR 8831, Mar. 19, 1987, as amended at 52 FR 23031, June 17, 1987; 55 FR 11579, Mar. 29, 1990; 57 FR 13249, Apr. 15, 1992]

Sec. 312.45 Inactive status.

a. If no subjects are entered into clinical studies for a period of 2 years or more under an IND, or if all investigations under an IND remain on clinical hold for 1 year or more, the IND may be placed by FDA on inactive status. This action may be taken by FDA either on request of the sponsor or on FDA's own initiative. If FDA seeks to act on its own initiative under this section, it shall first notify the sponsor in writing of the proposed inactive status. Upon receipt of such notification, the sponsor shall have 30 days to respond as to why the IND should continue to remain active.

b. If an IND is placed on inactive status, all investigators shall be so notified and all stocks of the drug shall be returned or otherwise disposed of in accordance with Sec. 312.59.

c. A sponsor is not required to submit annual reports to an IND on inactive status. An inactive IND is, however, still in effect for purposes of the public disclosure of data and information under Sec. 312.130.

d. A sponsor who intends to resume clinical investigation under an IND placed on inactive status shall submit a protocol amendment under Sec. 312.30 containing the proposed general investigational plan for the coming year and appropriate protocols. If the protocol amendment relies on information previously submitted, the plan shall reference such information. Additional information supporting the proposed investigation, if any, shall be submitted in an information amendment. Notwithstanding the provisions of Sec. 312.30, clinical investigations under an IND on inactive status may only resume (1) 30 days after FDA receives the protocol amendment, unless FDA notifies the sponsor that the investigations described in the amendment are subject to a clinical hold under Sec. 312.42, or (2) on earlier notification by FDA that the clinical investigations described in the protocol amendment may begin.

e. An IND that remains on inactive status for 5 years or more may be terminated under Sec. 312.44.

    (Collection of information requirements approved by the Office of Management and Budget under control number 0910-0014)

    [52 FR 8831, Mar. 19, 1987, as amended at 52 FR 23031, June 17, 1987]

Sec. 312.47 Meetings.

a. *General.* Meetings between a sponsor and the agency are frequently useful in resolving questions and issues raised during the course of a clinical investigation. FDA encourages such meetings to the extent that they aid in the evaluation of the drug and in the solution of scientific problems concerning the drug, to the extent that FDA's resources permit. The general principle underlying the conduct of such meetings is that there should be free, full, and open communication about any scientific or medical question that may arise during the clinical investigation. These meetings shall be conducted and documented in accordance with part 10.

b. "End-of-Phase 2" meetings and meetings held before submission of a marketing application. At specific times during the drug investigation process, meetings between FDA and a sponsor can be especially helpful in minimizing wasteful expenditures of time andmoney and thus in speeding the drug development and evaluation process. In particular, FDA has found that meetings at the end of Phase 2 of an investigation (end-of-Phase 2 meetings) are of considerable assistance in planning later studies and that meetings held near completion of Phase 3 and before submission of a marketing application ("pre-NDA" meetings) are helpful in developing methods of presentation and submission of data in the marketing application that facilitate review and allow timely FDA response.

1. End-of-Phase 2 meetings –

    i. Purpose. The purpose of an end-of-Phase 2 meeting is to determine the safety of proceeding to Phase 3, to evaluate the Phase 3 plan and protocols, and to identify any additional information necessary to support a marketing application for the uses under investigation.

    ii. Eligibility for meeting. While the end-of-Phase 2 meeting is designed primarily for IND's involving new molecular entities or major new uses of marketed drugs, a sponsor of any IND may request and obtain an end-of-Phase 2 meeting.

    iii. Timing. To be most useful to the sponsor, end-of-Phase 2 meetings should be held before major commitments of effort and resources to specific Phase 3 tests are made. The scheduling of an end-of-Phase 2 meeting is not, however, intended to delay the transition of an investigation from Phase 2 to Phase 3.

    iv. Advance information. At least 1 month in advance of an end-of-Phase 2 meeting, the sponsor should submit background information on the sponsor's plan for Phase 3, including summaries of the Phase 1 and 2 investigations, the specific protocols for Phase 3 clinical studies, plans for any additional nonclinical studies, and, if available, tentative labeling for the drug. The recommended contents of such a submission are described more fully in FDA Staff Manual Guide 4850.7 that is publicly available under FDA's public information regulations in part 20.

    v. Conduct of meeting. Arrangements for an end-of-Phase 2 meeting are to be made with the division in FDA's Center for Drug Evaluation and Research or the Center for Biologics Evaluation and Research which is responsible for review of the IND. The meeting will be scheduled by FDA at a time convenient to both FDA and the sponsor. Both the sponsor and FDA may bring consultants to the meeting. The meeting should be directed primarily at establishing agreement between FDA and the sponsor of the overall plan for Phase 3 and the objectives and design of particular studies. The adequacy of technical information to support Phase 3 studies and/or a marketing application may also be discussed. Agreements reached at the meeting on these matters will be recorded in minutes of the conference that will be taken by FDA in accordance with Sec. 10.65 and provided to the sponsor. The minutes along with any other written material provided to the sponsor will serve as a permanent record of any agreements reached. Barring a significant scientific development that requires otherwise, studies conducted in accordance with the agreement shall be presumed to be sufficient in objective and design for the purpose of obtaining marketing approval for the drug.

2. "Pre-NDA" meetings. FDA has found that delays associated with the initial review of a marketing application may be reduced by exchanges of information about a proposed marketing application. The primary purpose of this kind of exchange is to uncover any major unresolved problems, to identify those studies that the sponsor is relying on as adequate and well-controlled to establish the drug's effectiveness, to acquaint FDA reviewers with the general information to be submitted in the marketing application (including technical information), to discuss appropriate methods for statistical analysis of the data, and to discuss the best approach to the presentation and formatting of data in the marketing application. Arrangements for such a meeting are to be initiated by the sponsor with the division responsible for review of the IND. To permit FDA to provide the sponsor with the most useful advice on preparing a marketing application, the sponsor should submit to FDA's reviewing division at least 1 month in advance of the meeting the following information:

i. A brief summary of the clinical studies to be submitted in the application.

ii. A proposed format for organizing the submission, including methods for presenting the data.

iii. Any other information for discussion at the meeting.

(Collection of information requirements approved by the Office of Management and Budget under control number 0910-0014)

[52 FR 8831, Mar. 19, 1987, as amended at 52 FR 23031, June 17, 1987; 55 FR 11580, Mar. 29, 1990]

Sec. 312.48 Dispute resolution.

a. General. The Food and Drug Administration is committed to resolving differences between sponsors and FDA reviewing divisions withrespect to requirements for IND's as quickly and amicably as possible through the cooperative exchange of information and views.

b. Administrative and procedural issues. When administrative or procedural disputes arise, the sponsor should first attempt to resolve the matter with the division in FDA's Center for Drug Evaluation and Research or Center for Biologics Evaluation and Research which is responsible for review of the IND, beginning with the consumer safety officer assigned to the application. If the dispute is not resolved, the sponsor may raise the matter with the person designated as ombudsman, whose function shall be to investigate what has happened and to facilitate a timely and equitable resolution. Appropriate issues to raise with the ombudsman include resolving difficulties in scheduling meetings and obtaining timely replies to inquiries. Further details on this procedure are contained in FDA Staff Manual Guide 4820.7 that is publicly available under FDA's public information regulations in part 20.

c. Scientific and medical disputes.

   1. When scientific or medical disputes arise during the drug investigation process, sponsors should discuss the matter directly with the responsible reviewing officials. If necessary, sponsors may request a meeting with the appropriate reviewing officials and management representatives in order to seek a resolution. Requests for such meetings shall be directed to the director of the division in FDA's Center for Drug Evaluation and Research or Center for Biologics Evaluation and Research which is responsible for review of the IND. FDA will make every attempt to grant requests for meetings that involve important issues and that can be scheduled at mutually convenient times.

   2. The "end-of-Phase 2" and "pre-NDA" meetings described in Sec. 312.47(b) will also provide a timely forum for discussing and resolving scientific and medical issues on which the sponsor disagrees with the agency.

   3. In requesting a meeting designed to resolve a scientific or medical dispute, applicants may suggest that FDA seek the advice of outside experts, in which case FDA may, in its discretion, invite to the meeting one or more of its advisory committee members or other consultants, as designated by the agency. Applicants may rely on, and may bring to any meeting, their own consultants. For major scientific and medical policy issues not resolved by informal meetings, FDA may refer the matter to one of its standing advisory committees for its consideration and recommendations.

   [52 FR 8831, Mar. 19, 1987, as amended at 55 FR 11580, Mar. 29, 1990]

Subpart D – Responsibilities of Sponsors and Investigators

Sec. 312.50 General responsibilities of sponsors.

Sponsors are responsibile for selecting qualified investigators, providing them with the information they need to conduct an investigation properly, ensuring proper monitoring of the investigation(s), ensuring that the investigation(s) is conducted in accordance with the general investigational plan and protocols contained in the IND, maintaining an effective IND with respect to the investigations, and ensuring that FDA and all participating investigators are promptly informed of significant new adverse effects or risks with respect to the drug. Additional specific responsibilities of sponsors are described elsewhere in this part.

Sec. 312.52 Transfer of obligations to a contract research organization.

a. A sponsor may transfer responsibility for any or all of the obligations set forth in this part to a contract research organization. Any such transfer shall be described in writing. If not all obligations are transferred, the writing is required to describe each of the obligations being assumed by the contract research organization. If all obligations are transferred, a general statement that all obligations have been transferred is acceptable. Any obligation not covered by the written description shall be deemed not to have been transferred.

b. A contract research organization that assumes any obligation of a sponsor shall comply with the specific regulations in this chapter applicable to this obligation and shall be subject to the same regulatory action as a sponsor for failure to comply with any obligation assumed under these regulations. Thus, all references to "sponsor" in this part apply to a contract research organization to the extent that it assumes one or more obligations of the sponsor.

Sec. 312.53 Selecting investigators and monitors.

a. Selecting investigators. A sponsor shall select only investigators qualified by training and experience as appropriate experts to investigate the drug.

b. Control of drug. A sponsor shall ship investigational new drugs only to investigators participating in the investigation.

c. Obtaining information from the investigator. Before permitting an investigator to begin participation in an investigation, the sponsor shall obtain the following:

1. A signed investigator statement (Form FDA-1572) containing:
   i. The name and address of the investigator;
   ii. The name and code number, if any, of the protocol(s) in the IND identifying the study(ies) to be conducted by the investigator;
   iii. The name and address of any medical school, hospital, or other research facility where the clinical investigation(s) will be conducted;
   iv. The name and address of any clinical laboratory facilities to be used in the study;
   v. The name and address of the IRB that is responsible for review and approval of the study(ies);
   vi. A commitment by the investigator that he or she:

A. Will conduct the study(ies) in accordance with the relevant, current protocol(s) and will only make changes in a protocol after notifying the sponsor, except when necessary to protect the safety, the rights, or welfare of subjects;

B. Will comply with all requirements regarding the obligations of clinical investigators and all other pertinent requirements in this part;

C. Will personally conduct or supervise the described investigation(s);

D. Will inform any potential subjects that the drugs are being used for investigational purposes and will ensure that the requirements relating to obtaining informed consent (21 CFR part 50) and institutional review board review and approval (21 CFR part 56) are met;

E. Will report to the sponsor adverse experiences that occur in the course of the investigation(s) in accordance with Sec. 312.64;

F. Has read and understands the information in the investigator's brochure, including the potential risks and side effects of the drug; and

G. Will ensure that all associates, colleagues, and employees assisting in the conduct of the study(ies) are informed about their obligations in meeting the above commitments.

vii. A commitment by the investigator that, for an investigation subject to an institutional review requirement under part 56, an IRB that complies with the requirements of that part will be responsible for the initial and continuing review and approval of the clinical investigation and that the investigator will promptly report to the IRB all changes in the research activity and all unanticipated problems involving risks to human subjects or others, and will not make any changes in the research without IRB approval, except where necessary to eliminate apparent immediate hazards to the human subjects.

viii. A list of the names of the subinvestigators (e.g., research fellows, residents) who will be assisting the investigator in the conduct of the investigation(s).

2. Curriculum vitae. A curriculum vitae or other statement of qualifications of the investigator showing the education, training, and experience that qualifies the investigator as an expert in the clinical investigation of the drug for the use under investigation.

3. Clinical protocol.

   i. For Phase 1 investigations, a general outline of the planned investigation including the estimated duration of the study and the maximum number of subjects that will be involved.

   ii. For Phase 2 or 3 investigations, an outline of the study protocol including an approximation of the number of subjects to be treated with the drug and the number to be employed as controls, if any; the clinical uses to be investigated; characteristics of subjects by age, sex, and condition; the kind of clinical observations and laboratory tests to be conducted; the estimated duration of the study; and copies or a description of case report forms to be used.

4. Financial disclosure information. Sufficient accurate financial information to allow the sponsor to submit complete and accurate certification or disclosure statements required under part 54 of this chapter. The sponsor shall obtain a commitment from the clinical investigator to promptly update this information if any relevant changes occur during the course of the investigation and for 1 year following the completion of the study.

d. Selecting monitors. A sponsor shall select a monitor qualified by training and experience to monitor the progress of the investigation.
(Collection of information requirements approved by the Office of Management and Budget under control number 0910-0014)
[52 FR 8831, Mar. 19, 1987, as amended at 52 FR 23031, June 17, 1987; 61 FR 57280, Nov. 5, 1996; 63 FR 5252, Feb. 2, 1998]
Effective Date Note: At 63 FR 5252, Feb. 2, 1998, Sec. 312.53 was amended by adding new paragraph (c)(4), effective Feb. 2, 1999.

Sec. 312.54 Emergency research under Sec. 50.24 of this chapter.

a. The sponsor shall monitor the progress of all investigations involving an exception from informed consent under Sec. 50.24 of this chapter. When the sponsor receives from the IRB information concerning the public disclosures required by Sec. 50.24(a)(7)(ii) and (a)(7)(iii) of this chapter, the sponsor promptly shall submit to the IND file and to Docket Number 95S-0158 in the Dockets Management Branch (HFA-305), Food and Drug Administration, 12420 Parklawn Dr., rm. 1-23, Rockville, MD 20857, copies of the information that was disclosed, identified by the IND number.

b. The sponsor also shall monitor such investigations to identify when an IRB determines that it cannot approve the research because it does not meet the criteria in the exception in Sec. 50.24(a) of this chapter or because of other relevant ethical concerns. The sponsor promptly shall provide this information in writing to FDA, investigators who are asked to participate in this or a substantially equivalent clinical investigation, and other IRB's that are asked to review this or a substantially equivalent investigation.
[61 FR 51530, Oct. 2, 1996]

Sec. 312.55 Informing investigators.

a. Before the investigation begins, a sponsor (other than a sponsor-investigator) shall give each participating clinical investigator an investigator brochure containing the information described in Sec. 312.23(a)(5).

b. The sponsor shall, as the overall investigation proceeds, keep each participating investigator informed of new observations discovered by or reported to the sponsor on the drug, particularly with respect to adverse effects and safe use. Such information may be distributed to investigators by means of periodically revised investigator brochures, reprints or published studies, reports or letters to clinical investigators, or other appropriate means.Important safety information is required to be relayed to investigators in accordance with Sec. 312.32.

    (Collection of information requirements approved by the Office of Management and Budget under control number 0910-0014)

    [52 FR 8831, Mar. 19, 1987, as amended at 52 FR 23031, June 17, 1987]

Sec. 312.56 Review of ongoing investigations.

a. The sponsor shall monitor the progress of all clinical investigations being conducted under its IND.

b. A sponsor who discovers that an investigator is not complying with the signed agreement (Form FDA-1572), the general investigational plan, or the requirements of this part or other applicable parts shall promptly either secure compliance or discontinue shipments of the investigational new drug to the investigator and end the investigator's participation in the investigation. If the investigator's participation in the investigation is ended, the sponsor shall require that the investigator dispose of or return the investigational drug in accordance with the requirements of Sec. 312.59 and shall notify FDA.

c. The sponsor shall review and evaluate the evidence relating to the safety and effectiveness of the drug as it is obtained from the investigator. The sponsors shall make such reports to FDA regarding information relevant to the safety of the drug as are required under Sec. 312.32. The sponsor shall make annual reports on the progress of the investigation in accordance with Sec. 312.33.

d. A sponsor who determines that its investigational drug presents an unreasonable and significant risk to subjects shall discontinue those investigations that present the risk, notify FDA, all institutional review boards, and all investigators who have at any time participated in the investigation of the discontinuance, assure the disposition of all stocks of the drug outstanding as required by Sec. 312.59, and furnish FDA with a full report of the sponsor's actions. The sponsor shall discontinue the investigation as soon as possible, and in no event later than 5 working days after making the determination that the investigation should be discontinued. Upon request, FDA will confer with a sponsor on the need to discontinue an investigation.

(Collection of information requirements approved by the Office of Management and Budget under control number 0910-0014)

[52 FR 8831, Mar. 19, 1987, as amended at 52 FR 23031, June 17, 1987]

Sec. 312.57 Recordkeeping and record retention.

a. A sponsor shall maintain adequate records showing the receipt, shipment, or other disposition of the investigational drug. These records are required to include, as appropriate, the name of the investigator to whom the drug is shipped, and the date, quantity, and batch or code mark of each such shipment.

b. A sponsor shall maintain complete and accurate records showing any financial interest in Sec. 54.4(a)(3)(i), (a)(3)(ii), (a)(3)(iii), and (a)(3)(iv) of this chapter paid to clinical investigators by the sponsor of the covered study. A sponsor shall also maintain complete and accurate records concerning all other financial interests of investigators subject to part 54 of this chapter.

c. A sponsor shall retain the records and reports required by this part for 2 years after a marketing application is approved for the drug; or, if an application is not approved for the drug, until 2 years after shipment and delivery of the drug for investigational use is discontinued and FDA has been so notified.

d. A sponsor shall retain reserve samples of any test article and reference standard identified in, and used in any of the bioequivalence or bioavailability studies described in, Sec. 320.38 or Sec. 320.63 of this chapter, and release the reserve samples to FDA upon request, in accordance with, and for the period specified in Sec. 320.38.

    (Collection of information requirements approved by the Office of Management and Budget under control number 0910-0014)

    [52 FR 8831, Mar. 19, 1987, as amended at 52 FR 23031, June 17, 1987; 58 FR 25926, Apr. 28, 1993; 63 FR 5252, Feb. 2, 1998]

    Effective Date Note: At 63 FR 5252, Feb. 2, 1998, Sec. 312.57 was amended by redesignating paragraphs (b) and (c) as paragraphs (c) and (d) and by adding a new paragraph (b), effective Feb. 2, 1999.

Sec. 312.58 Inspection of sponsor's records and reports.

a. FDA inspection. A sponsor shall upon request from any properly authorized officer or employee of the Food and Drug Administration, at reasonable times, permit such officer or employee to have access to and copy and verify any records and reports relating to a clinical investigation conducted under this part. Upon written request by FDA, the sponsor shall submit the records or reports (or copies of them) to FDA. The sponsor shall discontinue shipments of the drug to any investigator who has failed to maintain or make available records or reports of the investigation as required by this part.

b. Controlled substances. If an investigational new drug is a substance listed in any schedule of the Controlled Substances Act (21 U.S.C. 801; 21

CFR part 1308), records concerning shipment, delivery, receipt, and disposition of the drug, which are required to be kept under this part or other applicable parts of this chapter shall, upon the request of a properly authorized employee of the Drug Enforcement Administration of the U.S. Department of Justice, be made available by the investigator or sponsor to whom the request is made, for inspection and copying. In addition, the sponsor shall assure that adequate precautions are taken, including storage of the investigational drug in a securely locked, substantially constructed cabinet, or other securely locked, substantially constructed enclosure, access to which is limited, to prevent theft or diversion of the substance into illegal channels of distribution.

Sec. 312.59 Disposition of unused supply of investigational drug.

The sponsor shall assure the return of all unused supplies of the investigational drug from each individual investigator whose participation in the investigation is discontinued or terminated. The sponsor may authorize alternative disposition of unused supplies of the investigational drug provided this alternative disposition does not expose humans to risks from the drug. The sponsor shall maintain written records of any disposition of the drug in accordance with Sec. 312.57.

(Collection of information requirements approved by the Office of Management and Budget under control number 0910-0014)

[52 FR 8831, Mar. 19, 1987, as amended at 52 FR 23031, June 17, 1987]

Sec. 312.60 General responsibilities of investigators.

An investigator is responsible for ensuring that an investigation is conducted according to the signed investigator statement, the investigational plan, and applicable regulations; for protecting the rights, safety, and welfare of subjects under the investigator's care; and for the control of drugs under investigation. An investigator shall, in accordance with the provisions of part 50 of this chapter, obtain the informed consent of each human subject to whom the drug is administered, except as provided in Secs. 50.23 or 50.24 of this chapter. Additional specific responsibilities of clinical investigators are set forth in this part and in parts 50 and 56 of this chapter.

[52 FR 8831, Mar. 19, 1987, as amended at 61 FR 51530, Oct. 2, 1996]

Sec. 312.61 Control of the investigational drug.

An investigator shall administer the drug only to subjects under the investigator's personal supervision or under the supervision of a subinvestigator responsible to the investigator. The investigator shall not supply the investigational drug to any person not authorized under this part to receive it.

Sec. 312.62 Investigator recordkeeping and record retention.

a. Disposition of drug. An investigator is required to maintain adequate records of the disposition of the drug, including dates, quantity, and use by subjects. If the investigation is terminated, suspended, discontinued, or completed, the investigator shall return the unused supplies of the drug to the sponsor, or otherwise provide for disposition of the unused supplies of the drug under Sec. 312.59.

b. Case histories. An investigator is required to prepare and maintain adequate and accurate case histories that record all observations and other data pertinent to the investigation on each individual administered the investigational drug or employed as a control in the investigation. Case histories include the case report forms and supporting data including, for example, signed and dated consent forms and medical records including, for example, progress notes of the physician, the individual's hospital chart(s), and the nurses' notes. The case history for each individual shall document that informed consent was obtained prior to participation in the study.

c. Record retention. An investigator shall retain records required to be maintained under this part for a period of 2 years following the date a marketing application is approved for the drug for the indication for which it is being investigated; or, if no application is to be filed or if the application is not approved for such indication, until 2 years after the investigation is discontinued and FDA is notified.

(Collection of information requirements approved by the Office of Management and Budget under control number 0910-0014)

[52 FR 8831, Mar. 19, 1987, as amended at 52 FR 23031, June 17, 1987; 61 FR 57280, Nov. 5, 1996]

Sec. 312.64 Investigator reports.

a. Progress reports. The investigator shall furnish all reports to the sponsor of the drug who is responsible for collecting and evaluating the results obtained. The sponsor is required under Sec. 312.33 to submit annual reports to FDA on the progress of the clinical investigations.

b. Safety reports. An investigator shall promptly report to the sponsor any adverse effect that may reasonably be regarded as caused by, or probably caused by, the drug. If the adverse effect is alarming, the investigator shall report the adverse effect immediately.

c. Final report. An investigator shall provide the sponsor with an adequate report shortly after completion of the investigator's participation in the investigation.

d. Financial disclosure reports. The clinical investigator shall provide the sponsor with sufficient accurate financial information to allow an applicant to submit complete and accurate certification or disclosure statements as required under part 54 of this chapter. The clinical investigator shall promptly update this information if any relevant changes occur during the course of the investigation and for 1 year following the completion of the study.

(Collection of information requirements approved by the Office of Management and Budget under control number 0910-0014)

[52 FR 8831, Mar. 19, 1987, as amended at 52 FR 23031, June 17, 1987; 63 FR 5252, Feb. 2, 1998]

Effective Date Note: At 63 FR 5252, Feb. 2, 1998, Sec. 312.64 was amended by adding new paragraph (d), effective Feb. 2, 1999.

Sec. 312.66 Assurance of IRB review.

An investigator shall assure that an IRB that complies with the requirements set forth in part 56 will be responsible for the initial and continuing review and approval of the proposed clinical study. The investigator shall also assure that he or she will promptly report to the IRB all changes in the research activity and all unanticipated problems involving risk to human subjects or others, and that he or she will not make any changes in the research without IRB approval, except where necessary to eliminate apparent immediate hazards to human subjects.

(Collection of information requirements approved by the Office of Management and Budget under control number 0910-0014)

[52 FR 8831, Mar. 19, 1987, as amended at 52 FR 23031, June 17, 1987]

Sec. 312.68 Inspection of investigator's records and reports.

An investigator shall upon request from any properly authorized officer or employee of FDA, at reasonable times, permit such officer or employee to have access to, and copy and verify any records or reports made by the investigator pursuant to Sec. 312.62. The investigator is not required to divulge subject names unless the records of particular individuals require a more detailed study of the cases, or unless there is reason to believe that the records do not represent actual case studies, or do not represent actual results obtained.

Sec. 312.69 Handling of controlled substances.

If the investigational drug is subject to the Controlled Substances Act, the investigator shall take adequate precautions, including storage of the investigational drug in a securely locked, substantially constructed cabinet, or other securely locked, substantially constructed enclosure, access to which is limited, to prevent theft or diversion of the substance into illegal channels of distribution.

Sec. 312.70 Disqualification of a clinical investigator.

a. If FDA has information indicating that an investigator (including a sponsor-investigator) has repeatedly or deliberately failed to comply with the requirements of this part, part 50, or part 56 of this chapter, or has submitted to FDA or to the sponsor false information in any required report, the Center for Drug Evaluation and Research or the Center for Biologics Evaluation and Research will furnish the investigator written notice of the matter complained of and offer the investigator an opportunity to explain the matter in writing, or, at the option of the investigator, in an informal conference. If an explanation is offered but not accepted by the Center for Drug Evaluation and Research or the Center for Biologics Evaluation and Research, the investigator will be given an opportunity for a regulatory hearing under part 16 on the question of whether the investigator is entitled to receive investigational new drugs.

b. After evaluating all available information, including any explanation presented by the investigator, if the Commissioner determines that the investigator has repeatedly or deliberately failed to comply with the requirements of this part, part 50, or part 56 of this chapter, or has deliberately or repeatedly submitted false information to FDA or to the sponsor in any required report, the Commissioner will notify the investigator and the sponsor of any investigation in which the investigator has been named as a participant that the investigator is not entitled to receive investigational drugs. The notification will provide a statement of basis for such determination.

c. Each IND and each approved application submitted under part 314 containing data reported by an investigator who has been determined to be ineligible to receive investigational drugs will be examined to determine whether the investigator has submitted unreliable data that are essential to the continuation of the investigation or essential to the approval of any marketing application.

d. If the Commissioner determines, after the unreliable data submitted by the investigator are eliminated from consideration, that the data remaining are inadequate to support a conclusion that it is reasonably safe to continue the investigation, the Commissioner will notify the sponsor who shall have an opportunity for a regulatory hearing under part 16. If a danger to the public health exists, however, the Commissioner shall terminate the IND immediately and notify the sponsor of the determination. In such case, the sponsor shall have an opportunity for a regulatory hearing before FDA under part 16 on the question of whether the IND should be reinstated.

e. If the Commissioner determines, after the unreliable data submitted by the investigator are eliminated from consideration, that the continued approval of the drug product for which the data were submitted cannot be justified, the Commissioner will proceed to withdraw approval of the drug product in accordance with the applicable provisions of the act.

f. An investigator who has been determined to be ineligible to receive investigational drugs may be reinstated as eligible when the Commissioner determines that the investigator has presented adequate assurances that the investigator will employ investigatioal drugs solely in compliance with theprovisions of this part and of parts 50 and 56.

(Collection of information requirements approved by the Office of Management and Budget under control number 0910-0014)

[52 FR 8831, Mar. 19, 1987, as amended at 52 FR 23031, June 17, 1987; 55 FR 11580, Mar. 29, 1990; 62 FR 46876, Sept. 5, 1997]

Subpart E – Drugs Intended to Treat Life-threatening and Severely-debilitating Illnesses

Sec. 312.80 Purpose.
Authority: Secs. 501, 502, 503, 505, 506, 507, 701, 52 Stat. 1049-1053 as amended, 1055-1056 as amended, 55 Stat. 851, 59 Stat. 463 as amended (21 U.S.C. 351, 352, 353, 355, 356, 357, 371); sec. 351, 58 Stat. 702 as amended (42 U.S.C. 262); 21 CFR 5.10, 5.11.
Source: 53 FR 41523, Oct. 21, 1988, unless otherwise noted.

The purpose of this section is to establish procedures designed to expedite the development, evaluation, and marketing of new therapies intended to treat persons with life-threatening and severely-debilitating illnesses, especially where no satisfactory alternative therapy exists. As stated Sec. 314.105(c) of this chapter, while the statutory standards of safety and effectiveness apply to all drugs, the many kinds of drugs that are subject to them, and the wide range of uses for those drugs, demand flexibility in applying the standards. The Food and Drug Administration (FDA) has determined that it is appropriate to exercise the broadest flexibility in applying the statutory standards, while preserving appropriate guarantees for safety and effectiveness. These procedures reflect the recognition that physicians and patients are generally willing to accept greater risks or side effects from products that treat life-threatening and severely-debilitating illnesses, than they would accept from products that treat less serious illnesses. These procedures also reflect the recognition that the benefits of the drug need to be evaluated in light of the severity of the disease being treated. The procedure outlined in this section should be interpreted consistent with that purpose.

Sec. 312.81 Scope.
This section applies to new drug, antibiotic, and biological products that are being studied for their safety and effectiveness in treating life-threatening or severely-debilitating diseases.
a. For purposes of this section, the term "life-threatening" means:
   1. Diseases or conditions where the likelihood of death is high unless the course of the disease is interrupted; and
   2. Diseases or conditions with potentially fatal outcomes, where the end point of clinical trial analysis is survival.
b. For purposes of this section, the term "severely debilitating" means diseases or conditions that cause major irreversible morbidity.
c. Sponsors are encouraged to consult with FDA on the applicability of these procedures to specific products.

Sec. 312.82 Early consultation.
For products intended to treat life-threatening or severely-debilitating illnesses, sponsors may request to meet with FDA-reviewing officials early in

the drug development process to review and reach agreement on the design of necessary preclinical and clinical studies. Where appropriate, FDA will invite to such meetings one or more outside expert scientific consultants or advisory committee members. To the extent FDA resources permit, agency reviewing officials will honor requests for such meetings

a. Pre-investigational new drug (IND) meetings. Prior to the submission of the initial IND, the sponsor may request a meeting with FDA-reviewing officials. The primary purpose of this meeting is to review and reach agreement on the design of animal studies needed to initiate human testing. The meeting may also provide an opportunity for discussing the scope and design of phase 1 testing, and the best approach for presentation and formatting of data in the IND.

b. End-of-phase 1 meetings. When data from phase 1 clinical testing are available, the sponsor may again request a meeting with FDA-reviewing officials. The primary purpose of this meeting is to review and reach agreement on the design of phase 2 controlled clinicaltrials, with the goal that such testing will be adequate to provide sufficient data on the drug's safety and effectiveness to support a decision on its approvability for marketing. The procedures outlined in Sec. 312.47(b)(1) with respect to end-of-phase 2 conferences, including documentation of agreements reached, would also be used for end-of-phase 1 meetings.

Sec. 312.83 Treatment protocols.

If the preliminary analysis of phase 2 test results appears promising, FDA may ask the sponsor to submit a treatment protocol to be reviewed under the procedures and criteria listed in Secs. 312.34 and 312.35. Such a treatment protocol, if requested and granted, would normally remain in effect while the complete data necessary for a marketing application are being assembled by the sponsor and reviewed by FDA (unless grounds exist for clinical hold of ongoing protocols, as provided in Sec. 312.42(b)(3)(ii)).

Sec. 312.84 Risk-benefit analysis in review of marketing applications for drugs to treat life-threatening and severely-debilitating illnesses.

a. FDA's application of the statutory standards for marketing approval shall recognize the need for a medical risk-benefit judgment in making the final decision on approvability. As part of this evaluation, consistent with the statement of purpose in Sec. 312.80, FDA will consider whether the benefits of the drug outweigh the known and potential risks of the drug and the need to answer remaining questions about risks and benefits of the drug, taking into consideration the severity of the disease and the absence of satisfactory alternative therapy.

b. In making decisions on whether to grant marketing approval for products that have been the subject of an end-of-phase 1 meeting under Sec. 312.82, FDA will usually seek the advice of outside expert scientific consultants or advisory committees. Upon the filing of such a marketing application under Sec. 314.101 or part 601 of this chapter, FDA will notify the members of the relevant standing advisory committee of the application's filing and its availability for review.

c. If FDA concludes that the data presented are not sufficient for marketing approval, FDA will issue (for a drug) a not approvable letter pursuant to Sec. 314.120 of this chapter, or (for a biologic) a deficiencies letter consistent with the biological product licensing procedures. Such letter, in describing the deficiencies in the application, will address why the results of the research design agreed to under Sec. 312.82, or in subsequent meetings, have not provided sufficient evidence for marketing approval. Such letter will also describe any recommendations made by the advisory committee regarding the application.

d. Marketing applications submitted under the procedures contained in this section will be subject to the requirements and procedures contained in part 314 or part 600 of this chapter, as well as those in this subpart.

Sec. 312.85 Phase 4 studies.

Concurrent with marketing approval, FDA may seek agreement from the sponsor to conduct certain postmarketing (phase 4) studies to delineate additional information about the drug's risks, benefits, and optimal use. These studies could include, but would not be limited to, studying different doses or schedules of administration than were used in phase 2 studies, use of the drug in other patient populations or other stages of the disease, or use of the drug over a longer period of time.

Sec. 312.86 Focused FDA regulatory research.

At the discretion of the agency, FDA may undertake focused regulatory research on critical rate-limiting aspects of the preclinical, chemical/manufacturing, and clinical phases of drug development and evaluation. When initiated, FDA will undertake such research efforts as a means for meeting a public health need in facilitating the development of therapies to treat life-threatening or severely debilitating illnesses.

Sec. 312.87 Active monitoring of conduct and evaluation of clinical trials.

For drugs covered under this section, the Commissioner and other agency officials will monitor the progress of the conduct and evaluation of clinical trials and be involved in facilitating their appropriate progress.

Sec. 312.88 Safeguards for patient safety.

All of the safeguards incorporated within parts 50, 56, 312, 314, and 600 of this chapter designed to ensure the safety of clinical testing and the safety of products following marketing approval apply to drugs covered by this section. This includes the requirements for informed consent (part 50 of this chapter) and institutional review boards (part 56 of this chapter). These safeguards further include the review of animal studies prior to initial human testing (Sec. 312.23), and the monitoring of adverse drug experiences through the requirements of IND safety reports (Sec. 312.32), safety update reports during agency review of a marketing application (Sec. 314.50 of this chapter), and postmarketing adverse reaction reporting (Sec. 314.80 of this chapter).

Sec. 312.110 Import and export requirements.

a. Imports. An investigational new drug offered for import into the United States complies with the requirements of this part if it is subject to an IND that is in effect for it under Sec. 312.40 and:
   1. The consignee in the United States is the sponsor of the IND;
   2. the consignee is a qualified investigator named in the IND; or
   3. the consignee is the domestic agent of a foreign sponsor, is responsible for the control and distribution of the investigational drug, and the IND identifies the consignee and describes what, if any, actions the consignee will take with respect to the investigational drug.

b. Exports. An investigational new drug intended for export from the United States complies with the requirements of this part as follows:
   1. If an IND is in effect for the drug under Sec. 312.40 and each person who receives the drug is an investigator named in the application; or
   2. If FDA authorizes shipment of the drug for use in a clinical investigation. Authorization may be obtained as follows:
      i. Through submission to the International Affairs Staff (HFY-50), Associate Commissioner for Health Affairs, Food and Drug Administration, 5600 Fishers Lane, Rockville, MD 20857, of a written request from the person that seeks to export the drug. A request must provide adequate information about the drug to satisfy FDA that the drug is appropriate for the proposed investigational use in humans, that the drug will be used for investigational purposes only, and that the drug may be legally used by that consignee in the importing country for the proposed investigational use. The request shall specify the quantity of the drug to be shipped per shipment and the frequency of expected shipments. If FDA authorizes exportation under this paragraph, the agency shall concurrently notify the government of the importing country of such authorization.
      ii. Through submission to the International Affairs Staff (HFY-50), Associate Commissioner for Health Affairs, Food and Drug Administration, 5600 Fishers Lane, Rockville, MD 20857, of a formal request from an authorized official of the government of the country to which the drug is proposed to be shipped. A request must specify that the foreign government has adequate information about the drug and the proposed investigational use, that the drug will be used for investigational purposes only, and that the foreign government is satisfied that the drug may

legally be used by the intended consignee in that country. Such a request shall specify the quantity of drug to be shipped per shipment and the frequency of expected shipments.

   iii. Authorization to export an investigational drug under paragraph (b)(2)(i) or (ii) of this section may be revoked by FDA if the agency finds that the conditions underlying its authorization are not longer met.

3. This paragraph applies only where the drug is to be used for the purpose of clinical investigation.

4. This paragraph does not apply to the export of an antibiotic drug product shipped in accordance with the provisions of section 801(d) of the act.

5. This paragraph does not apply to the export of new drugs (including biological products) approved for export under section 802 of the act or section 351(h)(1)(A) of the Public Health Service Act. (Collection of information requirements approved by the Office of Management and Budget under control number 0910-0014)

[52 FR 8831, Mar. 19, 1987, as amended at 52 FR 23031, June 17, 1987]

Subpart F – Miscellaneous

Sec. 312.120 Foreign clinical studies not conducted under an IND.

a. Introduction. This section describes the criteria for acceptance by FDA of foreign clinical studies not conducted under an IND. In general, FDA accepts such studies provided they are well designed, well conducted, performed by qualified investigators, and conducted in accordance with ethical principles acceptable to the world community. Studies meeting these criteria may be utilized to support clinical investigations in the United States and/or marketing approval. Marketing approval of a new drug or antibiotic drug based solely on foreign clinical data is governed by Sec. 314.106.

b. Data submissions. A sponsor who wishes to rely on a foreign clinical study to support an IND or to support an application for marketing approval shall submit to FDA the following information:

1. A description of the investigator's qualifications;

2. A description of the research facilities;

3. A detailed summary of the protocol and results of the study, and, should FDA request, case records maintained by the investigator or additional background data such as hospital or other institutional records;

4. A description of the drug substance and drug product used in the study, including a description of components, formulation,

specifications, and bioavailability of the specific drug product used in the clinical study, if available; and

5. If the study is intended to support the effectiveness of a drug product, information showing that the study is adequate and well controlled under Sec. 314.126.

c. Conformance with ethical principles.

1. Foreign clinical research is required to have been conducted in accordance with the ethical principles stated in the "Declaration of Helsinki" (see paragraph (c)(4) of this section) or the laws and regulations of the country in which the research was conducted, whichever represents the greater protection of the individual.

2. For each foreign clinical study submitted under this section, the sponsor shall explain how the research conformed to the ethical principles contained in the "Declaration of Helsinki" or the foreign country's standards, whichever were used. If the foreign country's standards were used, the sponsor shall explain in detail how those standards differ from the "Declaration of Helsinki" and how they offer greater protection.

3. When the research has been approved by an independent review committee, the sponsor shall submit to FDA documentation of such review and approval, including the names and qualifications of the members of the committee. In this regard, a "review committee" means a committee composed of scientists and, where practicable, individuals who are otherwise qualified (e.g., other health professionals or laymen). The investigator may not vote on any aspect of the review of his or her protocol by a review committee.

4. The "Declaration of Helsinki" states as follows:

Recommendations Guiding Physicians in Biomedical Research Involving Human Subjects

Introduction

It is the mission of the physician to safeguard the health of the people. His or her knowledge and conscience are dedicated to the fulfillment of this mission. The Declaration of Geneva of the World Medical Association binds the physician with the words, "The health of my patient will be my first consideration," and the International Code of Medical Ethics declares that, "A physician shall act only in the patient's interest when providing medical carewhich might have the effect of weakening the physical and mental condition of the patient."

The purpose of biomedical research involving human subjects must be to improve diagnostic, therapeutic and prophylactic procedures and the understanding of the aetiology and pathogenesis of disease.

In current medical practice most diagnostic, therapeutic or pro-phylactic procedures involve hazards. This applies especially to bio-medical research. Medical progress is based on research which ulti-mately must rest in part on experimentation involving human sub-jects.In the field of biomedical research a fundamental distinction must be recognized between medical research in which the aim is essentially diagnostic or therapeutic for a patient, and medical research, the essential object of which is purely scientific and with-out implying direct diagnostic or therapeutic value to the person subjected to the research.

Special caution must be exercised in the conduct of research which may affect the environment, and the welfare of animals used for research must be respected.

Because it is essential that the results of laboratory experiments be applied to human beings to further scientific knowledge and to help suffering humanity, the World Medical Association has pre-pared the following recommendations as a guide to every physician in biomedical research involving human subjects. They should be kept under review in the future. It must be stressed that the stan-dards as drafted are only a guide to physicians all over the world. Physicians are not relieved from criminal, civil and ethical responsi-bilities under the laws of their own countries.

I. Basic Principles

1. Biomedical research involving human subjects must conform to generally accepted scientific principles and should be based on adequately performed laboratory and animal experimentation and on a thorough knowledge of the scientific literature.

2. The design and performance of each experimental procedure involving human subjects should be clearly formulated in an experimental protocol which should be transmitted for consid-eration, comment and guidance to a specially appointed com-mittee independent of the investigator and the sponsor provid-ed that this independent committee is in conformity with the laws and regulations of the country in which the research exper-iment is performed.

3. Biomedical research involving human subjects should be con-ducted only by scientifically qualified persons and under the supervision of a clinically competent medical person. The responsibility for the human subject must always rest with a medically qualified person and never rest on the subject of the research, even though the subject has given his or her consent.

4. Biomedical research involving human subjects cannot legiti-mately be carried out unless the importance of the objective is in proportion to the inherent risk to the subject.

5. Every biomedical research project involving human subjects should be preceded by careful assessment of predictable risks in comparison with foreseeable benefits to the subject or to others. Concern for the interests of the subject must always prevail over the interests of science and society.

6. The right of the research subject to safeguard his or her integrity must always be respected. Every precaution should be taken to respect the privacy of the subject and to minimize the impact of the study on the subject's physical and mental integrity and on the personality of the subject.

7. Physicians should abstain from engaging in research projects involving human subjects unless they are satisfied that the hazards involved are believed to be predictable. Physicians should cease any investigation if the hazards are found to outweigh the potential benefits.

8. In publication of the results of his or her research, the physician is obliged to preserve the accuracy of the results. Reports of experimentation not in accordance with the principles laid down in this Declaration should not be accepted for publication.

9. In any research on human beings, each potential subject must be adequately informed of the aims, methods, anticipated benefits and potential hazards of the study and the discomfort it may entail. He or she should be informed that he or she is at liberty to abstain from participation in the study and that he or she is free to withdraw his or her consent to participation at any time. The physician should then obtain the subject's freely-given informed consent, preferably in writing.

10. When obtaining informed consent for the research project the physician should be particularly cautious if the subject is in a dependent relationship to him or her or may consent under duress. In that case the informed consent should be obtained by a physician who is not engaged in the investigation and who is completely independent of this official relationship.

11. In case of legal incompetence, informed consent should be obtained from the legal guardian in accordance with national legislation. Where physical or mental incapacity makes it impossible to obtain informed consent, or when the subject is a minor, permission from the responsible relative replaces that of the subject in accordance with national legislation. Whenever the minor child is in fact able to give a consent, the minor's consent must beobtained in addition to the consent of the minor's legal guardian.

12. The research protocol should always contain a statement of the ethical considerations involved and should indicate that the principles enunciated in the present Declaration are complied with.

II. Medical Research Combined with Professional Care (Clinical Research)

1. In the treatment of the sick person, the physician must be free to use a new diagnostic and therapeutic measure, if in his or her judgment it offers hope of saving life, reestablishing health or alleviating suffering.

2. The potential benefits, hazards and discomfort of a new method should be weighed against the advantages of the best current diagnostic and therapeutic methods.

3. In any medical study, every patient – including those of a control group, if any – should be assured of the best proven diagnostic and therapeutic method.

4. The refusal of the patient to participate in a study must never interfere with the physician-patient relationship.

5. If the physician considers it essential not to obtain informed consent, the specific reasons for this proposal should be stated in the experimental protocol for transmission to the independent committee (I, 2).

6. The physician can combine medical research with professional care, the objective being the acquisition of new medical knowledge, only to the extent that medical research is justified by its potential diagnostic or therapeutic value for the patient.

III. Non-Therapeutic Biomedical Research Involving Human Subjects (Non- Clinical Biomedical Research)

1. In the purely scientific application of medical research carried out on a human being, it is the duty of the physician to remain the protector of the life and health of that person on whom biomedical research is being carried out.

2. The subjects should be volunteers – either healthy persons or patients for whom the experimental design is not related to the patient's illness.

3. The investigator or the investigating team should discontinue the research if in his/her or their judgment it may, if continued, be harmful to the individual.

4. In research on man, the interest of science and society should never take precedence over considerations related to the well-being of the subject.

   (Collection of information requirements approved by the Office of Management and Budget under control number 0910-0014)
   [52 FR 8831, Mar. 19, 1987, as amended at 52 FR 23031, June 17, 1987; 56 FR 22113, May 14, 1991]

Sec. 312.130 Availability for public disclosure of data and information in an IND.

a. The existence of an investigational new drug application will not be disclosed by FDA unless it has previously been publicly disclosed or acknowledged.

b. The availability for public disclosure of all data and information in an investigational new drug application for a new drug or antibiotic drug will be handled in accordance with the provisions established in Sec. 314.430 for the confidentiality of data and information in applications submitted in part 314. The availability for public disclosure of all data and information in an investigational new drug application for a biological product will be governed by the provisions of Secs. 601.50 and 601.51.

c. Notwithstanding the provisions of Sec. 314.430, FDA shall disclose upon request to an individual to whom an investigational new drug has been given a copy of any IND safety report relating to the use in the individual.

d. The availability of information required to be publicly disclosed for investigations involving an exception from informed consent under Sec. 50.24 of this chapter will be handled as follows: Persons wishing to request the publicly disclosable information in the IND that was required to be filed in Docket Number 95S-0158 in the Dockets Management Branch (HFA-305), Food and Drug Administration, 12420 Parklawn Dr., rm. 1-23, Rockville, MD 20857, shall submit a request under the Freedom of Information Act.

[52 FR 8831, Mar. 19, 1987. Redesignated at 53 FR 41523, Oct. 21, 1988, as amended at 61 FR 51530, Oct. 2, 1996]

Sec. 312.140 Address for correspondence.

a. Except as provided in paragraph (b) of this section, a sponsor shall send an initial IND submission to the Central Document Room, Center for Drug Evaluation and Research, Food and Drug Administration, Park Bldg., Rm. 214, 12420 Parklawn Dr., Rockville, MD 20852. On receiving the IND, FDA will inform the sponsor which one of the divisions in the Center for Drug Evaluation and Research or the Center for Biologics Evaluation and Research is responsible for the IND. Amendments, reports, and other correspondence relating to matters covered by the IND should be directed to the appropriate division. The outside wrapper of each submission shall state what is contained in the submission, for example, "IND Application", "Protocol Amendment", etc.

b. Applications for the products listed below should be submitted to the Division of Biological Investigational New Drugs (HFB-230), Center for Biologics Evaluation and Research, Food and Drug Administration, 8800 Rockville Pike, Bethesda, MD 20892.

1. Products subject to the licensing provisions of the Public Health Service Act of July 1, 1944 (58 Stat. 682, as amended (42 U.S.C. 201 et seq.)) or subject to part 600;
2. ingredients packaged together with containers intended for the collection, processing, or storage of blood or blood components;
3. urokinase products;
4. plasma volume expanders and hydroxyethyl starch for leukapheresis; and
5. coupled antibodies, i.e., products that consist of an antibody component coupled with a drug or radionuclide component in which both components provide a pharmacological effect but the biological component determines the site of action.

c. All correspondence relating to biological products for human use which are also radioactive drugs shall be submitted to the Division of Oncology and Radiopharmaceutical Drug Products (HFD-150), Center for Drug Evaluation and Research, Food and Drug Administration, 5600 Fishers Lane, Rockville, MD 20857, except that applications for coupled antibodies shall be submitted in accordance with paragraph (b) of this section.

d. All correspondence relating to export of an investigational drug under Sec. 312.110(b)(2) shall be submitted to the International Affairs Staff (HFY-50), Office of Health Affairs, Food and Drug Administration, 5600 Fishers Lane, Rockville, MD 20857.

(Collection of information requirements approved by the Office of Management and Budget under control number 0910-0014)

[52 FR 8831, Mar. 19, 1987, as amended at 52 FR 23031, June 17, 1987; 55 FR 11580, Mar. 29, 1990]

Sec. 312.145 Guidelines.

a. FDA has made available guidelines under Sec. 10.90(b) to help persons to comply with certain requirements of this part.

b. The Center for Drug Evaluation and Research and the Center for Biologics Evaluation and Research maintain lists of guidelines that apply to the Centers' regulations. The lists state how a person can obtain a copy of each guideline. A request for a copy of the lists should be directed to the CDER Executive Secretariat Staff (HFD-8), Center for Drug Evaluation and Research, Food and Drug Administration, 5600 Fishers Lane, Rockville, MD 20857, for drug products, and the Congressional, Consumer, and International Affairs Staff (HFB-142), Center for Biologics Evaluation and Research, Food and Drug Administration, 8800 Rockville Pike, Bethesda, MD 20892, for biological products.

[52 FR 8831, Mar. 19, 1987, as amended at 55 FR 11580, Mar. 29, 1990; 56 FR 3776, Jan. 31, 1991; 57 FR 10814, Mar. 31, 1992]

Subpart G – Drugs for Investigational Use in Laboratory Research Animals or In Vitro Tests

Sec. 312.160 Drugs for investigational use in laboratory research animals or in vitro tests.

a. Authorization to ship.
   1. i. A person may ship a drug intended solely for tests in vitro or in animals used only for laboratory research purposes if it is labeled as follows:

      CAUTION: Contains a new drug for investigational use only in laboratory research animals, or for tests in vitro. Not for use in humans.

      ii. A person may ship a biological product for investigational in vitro diagnostic use that is listed in Sec. 312.2(b)(2)(ii) if it is labeled as follows:

      CAUTION: Contains a biological product for investigational in vitro diagnostic tests only.

   2. A person shipping a drug under paragraph (a) of this section shall use due diligence to assure that the consignee is regularly engaged in conducting such tests and that the shipment ofthe new drug will actually be used for tests in vitro or in animals used only for laboratory research.

   3. A person who ships a drug under paragraph (a) of this section shall maintain adequate records showing the name and post office address of the expert to whom the drug is shipped and the date, quantity, and batch or code mark of each shipment and delivery. Records of shipments under paragraph (a)(1)(i) of this section are to be maintained for a period of 2 years after the shipment. Records and reports of data and shipments under paragraph (a)(1)(ii) of this section are to be maintained in accordance with Sec. 312.57(b). The person who ships the drug shall upon request from any properly authorized officer or employee of the Food and Drug Administration, at reasonable times, permit such officer or employee to have access to and copy and verify records required to be maintained under this section.

b. Termination of authorization to ship. FDA may terminate authorization to ship a drug under this section if it finds that:
   1. The sponsor of the investigation has failed to comply with any of the conditions for shipment established under this section; or
   2. The continuance of the investigation is unsafe or otherwise contrary to the public interest or the drug is used for purposes other than bona fide scientific investigation. FDA will notify the person shipping the drug of its finding and invite immediate correction. If correction is not immediately made, the person shall have an opportunity for a regulatory hearing before FDA pursuant to part 16.

c. Disposition of unused drug. The person who ships the drug under paragraph (a) of this section shall assure the return of all unused supplies of the drug from individual investigators whenever the investigation discontinues or the investigation is terminated. The person who ships the drug may authorize in writing alternative disposition of unused supplies of the drug provided this alternative disposition does not expose humans to risks from the drug, either directly or indirectly (e.g., through food-producing animals). The shipper shall maintain records of any alternative disposition.

(Collection of information requirements approved by the Office of Management and Budget under control number 0910-0014)

[52 FR 8831, Mar. 19, 1987, as amended at 52 FR 23031, June 17, 1987. Redesignated at 53 FR 41523, Oct. 21, 1988]

GLOSSARY

Adverse Drug Reaction (ADR)
An unintended reaction to a drug taken at doses normally used in man for prophylaxis, diagnosis, or therapy of disease, or for the modification of physiological function. In clinical trials, an ADR would include any injuries by overdosing, abuse/dependence, and unintended interactions with other medicinal products.

Adverse Event (AE)
A negative experience encountered by an individual during the course of a clinical trial, that is associated with the drug. An AE can include previously undetected symptoms, or the exacerbation of a pre-existing condition. When an AE has been determined to be related to the investigational product, it is considered an Adverse Drug Reaction.

Biologic
A virus, therapeutic serum, toxin, antitoxin, vaccine, blood, blood component or derivative, allergenic product, or analogous product applicable to the prevention, treatment or cure of diseases or injuries of man.

Biotechnology
Any technique that uses living organisms, or substances from organisms, biological systems, or processes to make or modify a product or process, to change plants or animals, or to develop micro-organisms for specific uses.

Blinding
The process through which one or more parties to a clinical trial are unaware of the treatment assignments. In a single-blinded study, usually the subjects are unaware of the treatment assignments. In a double-blinded study, both the subjects and the investigators are unaware of the treatment assignments. Also, in a double-blinded study, the monitors and sometimes the data analysts are unaware. "Blinded" studies are conducted to prevent the unintentional biases that can affect subject data when treatment assignments are known.

Case Report Form (CRF)
A record of pertinent information collected on each subject during a clinical trial, as outlined in the study protocol.

Clinical Investigation
A systematic study designed to evaluate a product (drug, device, or biologic) using human subjects, in the treatment, prevention, or diagnosis of a disease or condition, as determined by the product's benefits relative to its risks. Clinical investigations can only be conducted with the approval of the Food and Drug Administration (FDA).

Clinical Trial
Any investigation in human subjects intended to determine the clinical pharmacological, pharmacokinetic, and/or other pharmacodynamic effects of an investigational agent, and/or to identify any adverse reactions to an investigational agent to assess the agent's safety and efficacy.

Control Group
The comparison group of subjects who are not treated with the investigational agent. The subjects in this group may receive no therapy, a different therapy, or a placebo.

Data Management
The process of handling the data gathered during a clinical trial. May also refer to the department responsible for managing data entry and database generation and/or maintenance.

Declaration of Helsinki
A series of guidelines adopted by the 18th World Medical Assembly in Helsinki, Finland in 1964. Address ethical issues for physicians conducting biomedical research involving human subjects. Recommendations include the procedures required to ensure subject safety in clinical trials, including informed consent and Ethics Committee reviews.

Demographic Data
Refers to the characteristics of study participants, including sex, age, family medical history, and other characteristics relevant to the study in which they are enrolled.

Device
An instrument, apparatus, implement, machine, contrivance, implant, in vitro reagent, or other similar or related article, including any component, part or accessory, which is intended for use in the diagnosis, cure, treatment or prevention of disease. A device does not achieve its intended purpose through chemical action in the body and is not dependent upon being metabolized to achieve its purpose.

Double-Blind
The design of a study in which neither the investigator or the subject knows which medication (or placebo) the subject is receiving.

Drug
As defined by the Food, Drug and Cosmetic Act, drugs are "articles (other than food) intended for the use in the diagnosis, cure, mitigation, treatment, or prevention of disease in man or other animals, or to affect the structure or any function of the body of man or other animals."

Drug Product
A finished dosage form (e.g. table, capsule, or solution) that contains the active drug ingredient usually combined with inactive ingredients.

Effective Dose
The dose of an investigational agent that produces the outcome considered "effective," as defined in the study protocol. This could mean a cure of the disease in question or simply the mitigation of symptoms.

Efficacy
A product's ability to produce beneficial effects on the duration or course of a disease. Efficacy is measured by evaluating the clinical and statistical results of clinical tests.

Ethics Committee
An independent group of both medical and non-medical professionals who are responsible for verifying the integrity of a study and ensuring the safety, integrity, and human rights of the study participants.

Exclusion Criteria
Refers to the characteristics that would prevent a subject from participating in a clinical trial, as outlined in the study protocol.

Food and Drug Administration (FDA)

A U.S. government agency responsible for ensuring compliance with the Food, Drug, and Cosmetics Act of 1938. All drugs sold in the U.S. must receive marketing approval from the FDA.

Formulation

The mixture of chemicals and/or biological substances and excipients used to prepare dosage forms.

Generic Drug

A medicinal product with the same active ingredient, but not necessarily the same inactive ingredients as a brand-name drug. A generic drug may only be marketed after the original drug's patent has expired.

Good Clinical Practice (GCP)

The FDA has established regulations and guidelines that specify the responsibilities of sponsors, investigators, monitors, and IRBs involved in clinical drug testing. These regulations are meant to protect the safety, rights and welfare of the patients in addition to ensuring the accuracy of the collected study data.

In Vitro Testing

Non-clinical testing conducted in an artificial environment such as a test tube or culture medium.

In Vivo Testing

Testing conducted in living animal and human systems.

Informed Consent

The voluntary verification of a patient's willingness to participate in a clinical trial, along with the documentation thereof. This verification is requested only after complete, objective information has given about the trial, including an explanation of the study's objectives, potential benefits, and risks and inconveniences, alternative therapies available, and of the subject's rights and responsibilities in accordance with the current revision of the Declaration of Helsinki.

Institutional Review Board (IRB)

An independent group of professionals designated to review and approve the clinical protocol, informed consent forms, study advertisements, and patient brochures, to ensure that the study is safe and effective for human participation. It is also the IRB's responsibility to ensure that the study adheres to the FDA's regulations.

Investigational New Drug Application (IND)

The petition through which a drug sponsor requests the FDA to allow human testing of its drug product.

Investigator

A medical professional, usually a physician but may also be a nurse, pharmacist or other health care professional, under whose direction an investigational drug is administered or dispensed. A principal investigator is responsible for the overall conduct of the clinical trial at his/her site.

Longitudinal Study

A study conducted over a long period of time.

MedWatch Program

An FDA program designed to monitor adverse events (AE) from drugs marketed in the U.S. Through the MedWatch program, health professionals may report AEs voluntarily to the FDA. Drug manufacturers are required to report all AEs brought to their attention.

New Drug Application (NDA)

The compilation of all nonclinical, clinical, pharmacological, pharmacokinetic and stability information required about a drug by the FDA in order to approve the drug for marketing in the U.S.

Nuremberg Code

As a result of the medical experimentation conducted by Nazis during World War II, the U.S. Military Tribunal in Nuremberg in 1947 set forth a code of medical ethics for researchers conducting clinical trials. The code is designed to protect the safety and integrity of study participants.

Off Label

The unauthorized use of a drug for a purpose other than that approved of by the FDA.

Open-Label Study

A study in which all parties, (patient, physician and study coordinator) are informed of the drug and dose being administered. In an open-label study, none of the participants are given placebos. These are usually conducted with Phase I & II studies.

Orphan Drug

A designation of the FDA to indicate a therapy developed to treat a rare disease (one which afflicts a U.S. population of less than 200,000 people). Because there are few financial incentives for drug companies to develop therapies for diseases that afflict so few people, the U.S. government offers additional incentives to drug companies (i.e. tax advantages and extended marketing exclusivity) that develop these drugs.

Over-the-Counter (OTC)
Drugs available for purchase without a physician's prescription.

Pharmacoeconomics
The study of cost-benefit ratios of drugs with other therapies or with similar drugs. Pharmacoeconomic studies compare various treatment options in terms of their cost, both financial and quality-of-life. Also referred to as "outcomes research."

Phase I Study
The first of four phases of clinical trials, Phase I studies are designed to establish the effects of a new drug in humans. These studies are usually conducted on small populations of healthy humans to specifically determine a drug's toxicity, absorption, distribution and metabolism.

Phase II Study
After the successful completion of phase I trials, a drug is then tested for safety and efficacy in a slightly larger population of individuals who are afflicted with the disease or condition for which the drug was developed.

Phase III Study
The third and last pre-approval round of testing of a drug is conducted on large populations of afflicted patients. Phase III studies usually test the new drug in comparison with the standard therapy currently being used for the disease in question. The results of these trials usually provide the information that is included in the package insert and labeling.

Phase IV Study
After a drug has been approved by the FDA, phase IV studies are conducted to compare the drug to a competitor, explore additional patient populations, or to further study any adverse events.

Pivotal Study
Usually a phase III study which presents the data that the FDA uses to decide whether or not to approve a drug. A pivotal study will generally be well-controlled, randomized, of adequate size, and whenever possible, double-blind.

Placebo
An inactive substance designed to resemble the drug being tested. It is used as a control to rule out any psychological effects testing may present. Most well-designed studies include a control group which is unwittingly taking a placebo.

Pre-Clinical Testing
Before a drug may be tested on humans, pre-clinical studies must be conducted either in vitro but usually in vivo on animals to determine that the drug is safe.

Protocol
A detailed plan that sets forth the objectives, study design, and methodology for a clinical trial. A study protocol must be approved by an IRB before investigational drugs may be administered to humans.

Quality Assurance
Systems and procedures designed to ensure that a study is being performed in compliance with Good Clinical Practice (GCP) guidelines and that the data being generated is accurate.

Randomization
Study participants are usually assigned to groups in such a way that each participant has an equal chance of being assigned to each treatment (or control) group. Since randomization ensures that no specific criteria are used to assign any patients to a particular group, all the groups will be equally comparable.

Regulatory Affairs
In clinical trials, the department or function that is responsible for ensuring compliance with government regulations and interacts with the regulatory agencies. Each drug sponsor has a regulatory affairs department that manages the entire drug approval process.

Serious Adverse Event (SAE)
Any adverse event (AE) that is fatal, life-threatening, permanently disabling, or which results in hospitalization, initial or prolonged.

Standard Operating Procedure (SOP)
Official, detailed, written instructions for the management of clinical trials. SOPs ensure that all the functions and activities of a clinical trial are carried out in a consistent and efficient manner.

Standard Treatment
The currently accepted treatment or intervention considered to be effective in the treatment of a specific disease or condition.

Treatment IND
A method through which the FDA allows seriously ill patients with no acceptable therapeutic alternative to access promising investigational drugs still in clinical development. The drug must show "sufficient evidence of safety and effectiveness." In recent decades many AIDs patients have been able to access unapproved therapies through this program.

About CenterWatch

CenterWatch is a Boston-based publishing company that focuses on the clinical trials industry. We provide a variety of information services used by pharmaceutical and biotechnology companies, CROs, SMOs, and investigative sites involved in the management and conduct of clinical trials. CenterWatch also provides educational materials for clinical research professionals, health professionals and for health consumers. Some of our top publications and services are described below. For a comprehensive listing with detailed information about our publications and services, please visit our web site at *www.centerwatch.com*.

About Center for Clinical Research Practice (CCRP)

The Center for Clinical Research Practice (CCRP) is a division of CenterWatch that provides educational materials and programs focusing on regulatory requirements and on safe and ethical practices in clinical research. Investigators, coordinators, administrators, IRB members and staff, and other health professionals involved in the conduct and management of clinical research use CCRP's publications and services. For more information, please visit *www.ccrp.com*.

Our Commitment and Guarantee

CenterWatch publications and services offer the highest quality news and information available. Subscribers to the *CenterWatch Newsletter* receive sharp discounts on most other periodicals, books and directories. We offer sharp discounts on quantity subscriptions and orders. To learn more about our quantity orders, please contact us at (617) 856-5900.

If at any time a subscriber decides to cancel their subscription to a CenterWatch periodical, CenterWatch will refund the entire paid subscription.

Contact Information
Kenneth A. Getz, President & Publisher
kenneth.getz@centerwatch.com

Joan A. Kroll, Director of Marketing & Sales
joan.kroll@centerwatch.com

CenterWatch · 22 Thomson Place · Boston, MA 02210
Tel (617) 856-5900 · Fax (617) 856-5901 · www.centerwatch.com

Periodicals

CenterWatch
An award-winning monthly newsletter that provides pharmaceutical and biotechnology companies, CROs, SMOs, academic institutions, research centers and the investment community with in-depth business news, feature articles on trends, original research and analysis, as well as grant lead information for investigative sites.

CenterWatch Europe
A quarterly electronic newsletter dedicated to providing news, information and analyses on the clinical trials industry in the European Union. *CenterWatch Europe* presents in-depth stories, timely insights, original data and analyses on all aspects of the relationship between pharmaceutical companies, CROs and investigator sites.

CW Weekly
A weekly newsletter—available as a fax or in electronic format—that reports on the top stories and breaking news in the clinical trials industry. Each weekly newsletter includes business headlines, financial information, market intelligence, drug pipeline and clinical trial results from the prior week.

JobWatch
A web-based resource at *www.centerwatch.com*, complimented by a print publication, that provides a comprehensive listing of career and educational opportunities in the clinical trials industry, including a searchable resume database service and online CE and CME accredited learning modules. Companies use JobWatch regularly to identify qualified clinical research professionals and career and educational services.

Books and Directories

The Investigator's Guide to Clinical Research, 3rd edition
A 250-page, step-by-step resource filled with tips, instructions and insights for health professionals interested in conducting clinical trials. *The Investigator's Guide* is designed to help the novice clinical investigator get involved in conducting clinical trials. The guide is also a valuable resource for experienced investigative sites looking for ways to improve and increase their involvement and success in clinical research. Developed in accordance with ACCME, readers can apply for CME credits. An exam is provided online.

How to Grow Your Investigative Site: A Guide to Operating and Expanding a Successful Clinical Research Center
This 300-page book is an ideal resource for clinical investigators interested in expanding their clinical trials operations in order to establish a more successful and effective research enterprise. Written by Barry Miskin, M.D. and Ann Neuer, the book is filled with practical instructions, insights, tips and resources designed to assist investigators and study personnel in growing a viable and successful clinical research business. Readers can apply for CME credits. An exam is provided online.

Protecting Study Volunteers in Research
One of our top-selling publications, this manual is recommended by the National Institutes of Health, the Office of Health and Human Services and by the FDA. *Protecting Study Volunteers in Research* is a 250-page manual designed to assist clinical research professionals in providing the highest standards of safety and ethical treatment for their study volunteers. Written specifically for academic institutions and IRBs actively involved in clinical trials, the manual is also applicable to independent investigative sites. The book has been developed in accordance with the ACCME. Readers can apply for CME credits or Nursing Credit Hours. An exam is provided with each manual.

A Guide to Patient Recruitment:
Today's Best Practices and Proven Strategies
A 350-page book designed to help clinical research professionals involved in managing and conducting clinical trials, improve the effectiveness of their patient recruitment efforts. Written by Diana Anderson, Ph.D., with contributions from 15 industry experts and thought leaders, this guide offers real world, practical recruitment strategies and tactics. It is considered an invaluable resource for educating staff on ways to improve patient recruitment and retention.

The Research Professional's Guide to E-Clinical Trials
This 300-page book is designed to assist clinical research professionals in understanding, planning and implementing a wide variety of web-based technologies. The book presents comprehensive information in an easy-to-understand format designed for both sophisticated and novice professionals. Written by Rebecca Kush, Ph.D., with contributions from industry experts, this guide offers useful insights into current technologies and how sponsors, CROs and investigative sites will use them.

An Industry in Evolution, 3rd edition
A 250-page sourcebook providing extensive data and facts documenting clinical trial industry trends and benchmarked practices. The material—charts, statistics and analytical reports—is presented in a well organized and easy-to-reference format. This important and valuable resource is used for developing business strategies and plans, for preparing presentations and for conducting business and market intelligence.

CenterWatch Compilation Reports Series
A collection of comprehensive, in-depth features, original research and analyses and fact-based company/institution business and financial profiles, reports are now available on *Site Management Organizations*, *Academic Medical Centers*, and *Contract Research Organizations*. Spanning nearly 5 years of in-depth coverage and analyses, these reports provide valuable insights into company strategies, market dynamics and successful business practices. Ideal for business planning and for market intelligence/market research.

The 2002 CenterWatch Directory of the Clinical Trials Industry
A comprehensive directory with over 1,000 pages of contact information and detailed company profiles for a wide range of organizations and individuals involved in the clinical trials industry. Considered the authoritative reference resource to organizations involved in designing, managing, conducting and supporting clinical trials.

The Directory of Drugs in Clinical Trials, 2nd edition
A comprehensive compilation of new, leading-edge medications currently in research, this directory offers a glimpse at new and upcoming treatment options in Phase I-III clinical trials, plus Pediatric trials. The Directory provides easy reference information on more than 1,800 drugs in active clinical trials across a variety of medical conditions. Detailed profile information is provided on each drug listed.

Profiles of Service Providers on the CenterWatch
Clinical Trials Listing Service™
The CenterWatch web site (*www.centerwatch.com*) attracts tens of thousands of sponsor and CRO company representatives every month that are

looking for experienced CROs and investigative sites to manage and conduct their clinical trials. No registration is required. Sponsors and CROs use this online directory free of charge. The CenterWatch web site offers all contract service providers—both CROs and investigative sites—the opportunity to present more information than any other Internet-based service available. This service is an ideal way to secure new contracts and clinical grants.

Patient Education Services

Volunteering For A Clinical Trial

An easy-to-read, six-page patient education brochure designed for research centers to provide consistent, professional and unbiased educational information for their potential clinical study subjects. The brochure is IRB approved. Sponsors, CROs and investigative sites use this brochure to inform patients about participating in clinical trials. *Volunteering for a Clinical Trial* can be distributed in a variety of ways including direct mailings to patients, displayed in waiting rooms, or as handouts to guide discussions. The brochure can be customized with company logos and custom information.

A Word from Study Volunteers: Opinions and Experiences of Clinical Trial Participants

A straightforward and easy-to-read ten-page pamphlet that reviews the results of a survey conducted among more than 1,200 clinical research volunteers. This brochure presents first hand experiences from clinical trial volunteers. It offers valuable insights for anyone interested in participating in a clinical trial. The brochure can be customized with company logos and custom information.

The New Medical Therapies Report Series

Reports in the *New Medical Therapies* Series are concise and easy-to-read. They are filled with thorough and in-depth information on clinical trial activities and drugs in development for specific illnesses and medical conditions. Reports are updated every six to 12 months to maintain their timeliness. An invaluable resource for clinical research and healthcare professionals interested in educating their patients about clinical trials, as well as for consumers and patients interested in staying informed about new and promising treatments being developed for their specific illness or medical condition. Reports are available in: Prostate Cancer, Depression, HIV/AIDS, Breast Cancer, Migraine, Lung Cancer, Alzheimer's disease, Colorectal Cancer, Melanoma, Hypertension/Heart Disease and Rheumatoid Arthritis/Osteoporosis. Please visit our web site, *www.centerwatch.com* for a listing of additional reports available.

*Informed Consent: The Consumer's Guide to
the Risks and Benefits of Volunteering for a Clinical Trial*
A must-read paperback book for patients and health consumers currently involved in a clinical trial or evaluating whether to participate. This valuable resource provides a wealth of facts, insights and case examples designed to assist individuals in making informed decisions about including clinical trials among their treatment options.

The CenterWatch Clinical Trials Listing Service™
Now in its sixth year of operation, *The CenterWatch Clinical Trials Listing Service™* provides the largest and most comprehensive listing of Industry and Government-sponsored clinical trials on the Internet. In 2002, the CenterWatch web site—along with numerous coordinated online and print affiliations—is expected to reach more than 5 million Americans. *The CenterWatch Clinical Trials Listing Service™* provides an international listing of more than 40,000 ongoing and IRB-approved phase I–IV clinical trials.

Information Services

Research Reports and Custom Market Research Services
The CenterWatch Market Research team conducts custom projects designed to assist companies in answering a variety of mission critical issues that relate to their clinical trial operations and new strategy formation. The CenterWatch staff brings unprecedented expertise in gathering and analyzing information about all aspects of the clinical trials industry. CenterWatch clients include major pharmaceutical and biotechnology companies, CROs, investigative sites, investment banks and management consulting firms.

TrialWatch Site-Identification Service
Several hundred sponsor and CRO companies use the TrialWatch service to identify prospective investigative sites to conduct their upcoming clinical trials. Every month, companies post bulletins of their phase I-IV development programs that are actively seeking clinical investigators. These bulletins are included in the *CenterWatch Newsletter*—our flagship publication that reaches as many as 30,000 experienced investigators every month. Use of the TrialWatch service is FREE.

Content License Services
CenterWatch offers both database content and static text under license. All CenterWatch content can be seamlessly integrated into your company Internet, Intranet or Extranet web site(s) with or without frames. Our database offerings include: the *Clinical Trials Listing Service™*, *Clinical Trial Results, Drugs in Clinical Trials, Newly Approved Drugs, The Clinical Trial Industry Directory,* and *CW-Mobile* for Wireless OS® Devices. Our static text offerings include: an editorial feature on background information on

Clinical Trials, a *Glossary of Clinical Trial terminology*, and *New Medical Therapies Reports*.

Center for Clinical Research Practice Publications and Services

Training and Education Publications

Research Practitioner
Award winning bi-monthly journal with articles and features covering regulatory developments and trends, issues in clinical research management, drug and device development, protocol design, and implementation, and other topics germane to clinical research professionals. Continuing medical education credit (CME) is available through Boston University School of Medicine. Continuing education in nursing through ANCC provider.

Foundations of Clinical Research
An independent study course for health professionals involved in the management and conduct of clinical trials. This course provides a solid introduction to research practice today from the historical roots of biomedical experimentation through protocol design, implementation and management, this course provides a solid introduction to research practice today. Continuing education credit for nurses and physicians is available. Includes a Textbook, Workbook, Answer Key, Sample Protocol and CE Test. A perfect resource for new or moderately experienced members of the research staff at investigative sites, SMOs, Sponsors, and CROs. Currently used as the training curriculum at large academic institutions and universities.

Foundations of Human Subject Protection
An independent study course that covers the basic ethical concepts and regulatory requirements of human subject research. This course will teach you how to conduct clinical research in an ethical and scientific manner and know how to apply sound ethical judgment. Specifically written for IRB members, staff, clinical researchers and healthcare professionals involved in the conduct and management of clinical research. Continuing education credit for nurses and physicians is available. Includes a Textbook and CE Test.

Research Management Publications

STANDARD OPERATING PROCEDURES (SOPs)
FOR SPONSORS, SITES AND IRBs

Standard Operating Procedures for Good Clinical Practice by Sponsors
Template SOPs based on the ICH/GCP Consolidated Guidelines and the
Code of Federal Regulations and is pertinent to the development, initiation,
conduct and oversight of clinical research. The printed template is provided
in a 3-ring binder and on CD-ROM for installation on your Company's
computer or intranet. This comprehensive document covers the regulatory
requirements, including: document control (SOP, controlled documents,
forms); FDA and NIH contacts and submissions (IND, IDE, reports, gene
therapy), project management (communication, investigational product
inventory); monitoring visits and reports, human subject protection (IRB,
consent); data handling (CRF completion, electronic systems); quality
assurance (site audits, FDA inspections) and more. An essential document
for FDA-regulated drug and device studies and for federally-sponsored
research for Sponsors and Sponsor-Investigators holding INDs/IDEs.

Standard Operating Procedures for Good Clinical Practice
at the Investigative Site
Template SOPs based on the ICH/GCP Consolidated Guidelines and the
Code of Federal Regulations and is pertinent to the day-to-day conduct of
clinical research and is designed to be customized for your research facility.
This easy-to-use template is provided in a 3-ring binder and on 2 diskettes
(in Word 95/97) for installation on your computer. Use *Standard Operating*
Procedures for Good Clinical Practice at the Investigative Site to showcase your
site's blueprint for compliance and to highlight your critical standards valued by Sponsors, CROs and your research team.

Policies and Standard Operating Procedures
for the Institutional Review Board (IRB)
Template SOPs for IRBs that primarily review biomedical research. The
policies and procedures are based on regulatory requirements, ethical principles, and ICH guidelines and include the tools and information that IRB
staff need to conduct the day-to-day activities of the IRB office. It is provided as a written document and on CD-ROM for installation of the IRBs computer system.

Regulatory References
A handy and comprehensive compilation of the federal regulations, guidance documents, and principles that form the basis of how clinical trials are
conducted. A 297-page manual with CD-ROM comes in 2 Versions—for
Sponsors or investigative sites and IRBs (includes OHRP IRB Guidebook
and FDA IRB self audit). It is available in Word for Windows, is fully search-

able with "cut & paste" function for internal use. A great companion document for SOPs.

Institutional Review Board Services

New England Institutional Review Board (NEIRB)
NEIRB serves as an ethical review board for multi-site studies and individual researchers for industry and government-sponsored clinical trials of drugs, biologics, and devices. Founded twelve years ago, NEIRB is comprised of highly qualified members with significant experience and knowledge in the scientific, legal and ethical aspects of clinical trials. A professional and responsive administrative staff is focused on client service.

The NEIRB is managed and operated under all applicable regulations and Good Clinical Practice Guidelines from the International Conference on Harmonisation. NEIRB has been audited by the United States Food and Drug Administration and found to be in compliance with regulations. NEIRB is affiliated with the Commonwealth of Massachusetts, Department of Public Health, a requirement for reviewing research in Massachusetts and is, therefore, one of the only independent review boards able to review studies in all states.

About the Author

David Ginsberg, D.O., is a board-certified family practitioner, and is currently CEO and President of Omnicomm Systems, Inc., a web based company specializing in electronic data capture and transfer. Dr. Ginsberg previously was employed as Vice President of Field Operations at Wyeth-Ayerst, the research division of American Home Products. Prior to working for Wyeth-Ayerst, David was a practicing physician and principal investigator for more than 15 years. All in all, David has conducted more than 300 industry-sponsored clinical trials. David also created and ran site management organizations, independently and for integrated healthcare systems and managed care organizations. For two years, David worked for Covance, a top five contract research organization, where he was responsible for creating initiatives and interacting with investigators, integrated health systems and academic medical centers on a global basis.